Contents

Radcliffe Publishing Ltd
33–41 Dallington Street
London
EC1V 0BB
United Kingdom

www.radcliffepublishing.com

British Library Cataloguing in Publication Data

A catalogue record for this book is available from the British Library.

ISBN-13: 978 184619 516 7

The paper used for the text pages of this book is FSC® certified. FSC (The Forest Stewardship Council®) is an international network to promote responsible management of the world's forests.

MIX
Paper from
responsible sources
FSC
www.fsc.org   FSC® C013056

Typeset by Kate Broome, Auckland, New Zealand
Printed and bound by TJI Digital, Padstow, Cornwall, UK

Communication Skills in Mental Health Care

AN INTRODUCTION

Edited by

XAVIER COLL

Consultant Child and Adolescent Psychiatrist
Mary Chapman House, Norfolk and Suffolk NHS Foundation Trust
Honorary Senior Lecturer
School of Medicine, University of East Anglia, Norwich

ALEXIA PAPAGEORGIOU

Senior Lecturer in Clinical Communication
University of Nicosia's St George's (University of London) Medical Programme

ANN STANLEY

Consultant Forensic Psychiatrist
Norvic Clinic, Norfolk and Suffolk NHS Foundation Trust
Recognised Teacher
University of East Anglia, Norwich

and

ANDREW TARBUCK

Consultant in Old Age Psychiatry
Julian Hospital, Norfolk and Suffolk NHS Foundation Trust
Honorary Senior Lecturer
School of Medicine, University of East Anglia, Norwich

Foreword by

JONATHAN SILVERMAN

Associate Clinical Dean and Director of Communication Studies
School of Clinical Medicine
University of Cambridge

Radcliffe Publishing
London • New York

To our families, friends, colleagues, students and patients.

Foreword

Health care professionals working with patients with mental health issues face some of the most complex communication challenges in medicine. Consider for a moment the common problems that patients present with to both psychiatric services and primary care. Health professionals will be consulting with patients at risk of self-harm and suicide, who have disordered thought processes, who may be delusional or paranoid, with problems of capacity in old age or of confidentiality with young people. They will be routinely working with significant emotions or with patients with medically unexplained symptoms and will be dealing with distressed family members as well as the patient themselves. They will be working with patients with complex alcohol- and drug-related problems.

These challenges which might faze other medical practitioners will be the bread-and-butter of those working with patients with mental health issues. Communication will be all-important. Knowledge about psychiatric conditions is vital. But by itself without the communication process skills necessary to form a relationship, obtain appropriate complex and sensitive information, share decision making with the patient where possible or communicate where the health professional must make decisions against the patient's wishes, health care professionals will struggle to get the best out of the interview and achieve a satisfactory working life, and patients will not be supported in dealing with their mental health issues. Health care outcomes will suffer and health care practitioners may also.

Xavier Coll, Alexia Papageorgiou, Ann Stanley and Andrew Tarbuck have produced an important, highly readable and very well-organised account of how to organise mental health consultations. They look first at the general issues of the overall psychiatric history and then move onto the more complex specialist scenarios as outlined above. They have taken an approach which importantly integrates the content of the interview (the information that we are trying to obtain or impart), the process of the interview (the ways we communicate with patients; how we go about discovering the history or providing information, the verbal and non-verbal skills we use, how we develop the relationship with the patient, the way we organise and structure the interview) and the perceptual (the clinical reasoning and problem-solving skills that underlie the direction we take the interview).

The authors have chosen to use the Calgary–Cambridge model to provide a clear structure and skill set throughout the book. As one of the authors of the approach,

I'm delighted to see our work so carefully mapped onto the daily life of health care professionals. Interestingly, when we wrote our approach, we said the following:

> 'The skills collated in the guides provide the foundations for effective doctor–patient communication in a variety of different medical contexts. There are many highly challenging situations for doctors when they communicate with patients, such as in breaking bad news, bereavement, revealing hidden depression, gender and cultural issues, communicating with older patients, prevention and motivation. These issues clearly deserve special attention in our teaching and we shall be exploring them further. However, we stress that the skills delineated in the guides are the <u>core</u> communication skills required in all these circumstances, providing a secure platform for tackling these specific communication issues. Although the context of the interaction changes and the content of the communication varies, the process skills themselves remain the same: the challenge is to deepen our understanding of these core skills and the level of mastery with which we apply them.'

This book does just what we were recommending. It takes the core skills of the guide and shows how they apply in different circumstances in complex consultations. Each issue is approached using the same structure and skill sets. Yet on each occasion, how to operationalise the skills is covered in detail so the reader can see how to selectively, skilfully and deliberately apply the skills in different contexts. We had intended the skills to be used flexibly and not slavishly depending on the context. This book demonstrates just how to use the skills intentionally in different situations and considers whether indeed they may have to be carefully modified such as in the reversal of the open to closed cone in patients with psychosis.

What is particularly valuable is the amount of specific examples of phrasing included in the text to give readers a sense of how to accomplish these tasks from a communication process perspective. The message rings out that the clinicians writing each chapter have not only immense practical experience of the situations that they are describing but also have thought very carefully about the communication skills necessary to accomplish their goals.

I'm delighted to recommend this text and congratulate the editors and contributors on their contribution to the extremely important field of communicating in mental health care.

Jonathan Silverman
Associate Clinical Dean and Director of Communication Studies
School of Clinical Medicine
University of Cambridge
January 2012

Preface

Effective communication skills are the essence of good health-care practice. Health-care professionals with effective communication skills receive fewer complaints from patients and their relatives. They also carry out more efficient consultations, enjoy a more satisfactory working life and produce improved patient health outcomes. This book provides a clear and concise guide on how to run consultations using the Calgary–Cambridge model, as applied to a range of mental health conditions, ranging from taking a good psychiatric history to specialist scenarios, such as working with families and young people or breaking bad news in mental health, as well as chapters on anxiety, depression, psychosis, risk to self, mental capacity, dealing with emotions and mental health consultations in primary care. This book includes a DVD in which the authors have enacted the answers to the OSCE practice tasks that are formulated at the end of each chapter, to support the OSCEs model answers from Appendix 7.

XC, AP, AS and AT
January 2012

About this book

The chapters of this book should be able to stand alone and be read as one needs them. Having said this, for the newcomers to mental health, we would recommend initially reading Chapter 2, taking a good psychiatric history, first, to firmly set the foundations.

About the editors

Dr Xavier Coll is a Consultant Child and Adolescent Psychiatrist at the Norfolk and Suffolk NHS Foundation Trust and an Honorary Senior Lecturer at the School of Medicine of the University of East Anglia (UEA), in Norwich, UK. Dr Coll graduated from the Medical School of the Universitat Autònoma of Barcelona, in Spain, training in psychiatry in Bath, North Devon, Oxford and Southampton. His PhD focused on the experiences of abuse that women who deliberately harmed themselves had suffered. The interviews with them raised Xavier's awareness of the communication challenges faced by both clinicians and patients. He has been involved with the UEA since his arrival in Norwich in 1999, where he is an Educational and Clinical Supervisor, a Problem Based Learning (PBL) Tutor, Communication Skills Tutor and Examiner, as well as being part of a small team that organises and develops the mental health component of the curriculum. He enjoys listening to and playing music, sports (especially tennis, basketball and football), reading, and communicating with people when he travels. He hopes you will enjoy this book and find it helpful, practical and informative.

Dr Alexia Papageorgiou is a Senior Lecturer in Clinical Communication at the University of Nicosia's St George's (University of London) Medical Programme. Between 2003 and 2011, she worked for the University of East Anglia, in Norwich, UK where she designed and facilitated the implementation of the communication skills course for the undergraduate medical curriculum. During this time, she served as a member of the UK Council of Clinical Communication in Undergraduate Medical Education. She has extensive knowledge and experience in mental health settings, as she worked in therapeutic communities for chronically mentally ill people between 1990 and 1997. Her PhD in psychiatry focused on psychiatric advance statements designed by sectioned patients, which gave her further insight into the communication challenges faced by both mental health professionals and patients. She enjoys cooking, reading, swimming, cycling and walking.

Dr Ann Stanley, Consultant Forensic Psychiatrist, Norfolk and Suffolk NHS Foundation Trust and University of East Anglia, Norvic Clinic, St Andrew's

Business Park, Norwich, UK. Dr Stanley graduated from the University of London (Royal Free Hospital Medical School) in 1986. She undertook her psychiatric training in Birmingham. She has worked in Norwich since 1998, having been involved with UEA since the start of the medical course. She is an OSCE Examiner as well as teaching communication skills. One of her interests is the representation of mental illness in fiction and how it has changed over time; other interests are art, cooking and sewing.

Dr Andrew Tarbuck has been a Consultant in Old Age Psychiatry at the Julian Hospital, Norwich, since 1995, and has been the Director of the DeNDRoN (Dementias & Neurodegenerative Diseases) Local Research Network in East Anglia since 2006. He is an Honorary Senior Lecturer at the University of East Anglia and has been closely involved in curriculum development, teaching and examining of medical students. Dr Tarbuck read medicine at Gonville and Caius College, Cambridge and Green College, Oxford. He trained in psychiatry at Fulbourn Hospital, Cambridge and St Andrew's Hospital, Norwich. Outside work, his interests include gardening, life drawing, sculpture and taking a scruffy and disobedient West Highland white terrier for long walks in the Norfolk countryside.

List of contributors

Dr Jane Calne is a General Practitioner in Norfolk, a Practitioner in Rheumatology at the Norfolk and Norwich University Hospital, and a Senior Lecturer at the University of East Anglia's Medical School in Norwich, UK.

Dr Jaap Hamelijnk has been a Consultant in General Adult Psychiatry with the Norfolk and Suffolk NHS Foundation Trust since September 2001. He qualified from the University of Amsterdam Medical School in 1990. After training as a GP first, he completed psychiatry training in North Wales. He is based in Lowestoft, where he works with the Early Intervention in Psychosis Team for Waveney, also being the Primary Care Consultant for the Eating Disorders Team for Great Yarmouth and Waveney. Dr Hamelijnk runs a developmental disorder clinic for adults with ADHD and/or autistic spectrum conditions. He is also Communication Skills Tutor for the UEA's medical school in Norwich.

Dr Katherine Hill is a Consultant Psychiatrist practising at the Central Norfolk Early Intervention Team of the Norfolk and Suffolk NHS Foundation Trust.

Dr Rebecca Horne is a General Adult Psychiatrist working in a community mental health team based in Norwich. She trained in medicine at Charing Cross and Westminster Medical School, University of London. She completed her specialist training in psychiatry in the East Anglian region. Her interests include cognitive behavioural therapy, women's mental health and interfaces in psychiatry.

Dr Lisa Jackson is a General Practitioner at the East Norwich Medical Partnership and a Senior Lecturer at the Medical School in Norwich.

Dr Somayya Kajee is a Consultant in General Adult Psychiatry with the Norfolk and Suffolk NHS Foundation Trust. She is based in Lowestoft.

Dr Sarah Maxwell is a Consultant Child and Adolescent Psychiatrist at the Norfolk and Suffolk NHS Foundation Trust and an Honorary Senior Lecturer at the School of Medicine of the University of East Anglia (UEA), in Norwich. Dr Maxwell trained at both Oxford University and University College London. She has been involved with the UEA since becoming a Consultant in 2005, where she is a Consultation Skills Tutor and OSCE Examiner. Dr Maxwell is interested in travelling and sailing, and is hoping to combine the two and sail around the world in her old age.

Dr Nick Viale is a Consultant in Old Age Psychiatry at the Norfolk and Suffolk NHS Foundation Trust and is based at the Julian Hospital, Norwich. Outside of work he enjoys a busy family life, running, playing badminton and reading.

Dr Roger Wesby is a Consultant Psychiatrist for Older Persons, and Psychotherapy Tutor in Norfolk and Suffolk NHS Foundation Trust, where he co-runs a two-year training module in advanced communication skills for core trainees in psychiatry. He is an Honorary Senior Lecturer at the University of East Anglia, where he teaches communication skills. He is a Jungian analyst and is registered with the British Psychoanalytic Council.

Dr Jonathan Wilson is a Consultant Psychiatrist and Psychotherapist working with the Early Intervention Service in Norwich, Norfolk. He is also Honorary Senior Lecturer at the University of East Anglia.

Acknowledgements

We would like to thank our authors for their contribution and expertise in producing this book as well as our students and communication skills tutors, who provided us with a wealth of experience in teaching this subject and paving the way for writing this book.

List of figures and tables

CHAPTER 1

Introduction

Alexia Papageorgiou

WHY ARE TEACHING AND LEARNING COMMUNICATION SKILLS IN MENTAL HEALTH IMPORTANT?

Mental illness presents a challenge in today's global and national health systems (Murray and Lopez, 1996; Jenkins *et al.*, 2003; Singleton *et al.*, 2003). According to the World Health Organization (WHO), severe mental illness, such as schizophrenia, bipolar affective disorder, schizo-affective disorder, clinical depression, and drug and alcohol misuse accounted for about 11% of the global burden of disease in 1990 and is expected to rise to 15% by 2020 (Murray and Lopez, 1996).

In Britain the 2001 census suggested that approximately one in six adults had been assessed as having a neurotic disorder, with the most prevalent neurotic disorders being mixed anxiety and depression (88 cases per 1000). These disorders were more prevalent in adults between 40 and 54 years of age. The prevalence of psychotic disorder in adults was approximately five per 1000 (Singleton *et al.*, 2003). Neurosis is associated with high morbidity, while severe mental illness (e.g. psychosis) is associated with both high mortality and morbidity and demands significant involvement of all health-care and community systems (e.g. primary/secondary care interface, workplaces and community settings) (Harris and Barraclough, 1998; Singleton *et al.*, 2003).

Moderate to severe mental illnesses are treated using a combination of drugs and psychological therapies. These can be addressed in primary care within the community and/or in specialist mental health services in secondary care. Whichever route is taken, the delivery of care is improved when the mental health consultation is done in a manner sensitive to the patient's condition. This has been shown to help the patient to engage more easily and maintain better contact with the services. When interacting with a patient exhibiting mental health issues, a clinician may well experience significant communication challenges. Such patients may demonstrate unpredictable mood swings, low self-esteem, dissociation from their surroundings, misinterpretation of communication and paranoia (Silverman *et al.*, 2005).

The effective communication skills necessary to develop rapport with such patients need to be developed by a combination of training and experience. To learn from experience alone is seldom as productive and always more time consuming. Lack of communication skills during these interactions can lead to patient resentfulness and detachment from services, resulting in a decline in mental health and the possibility of compulsory admission, and risk to self and others (Priebe *et al.*, 2005).

Research evidence suggests that both mental health care professionals and their patients experience a challenge in communicating about symptoms and drug treatments and their side effects. This hinders the goal of reaching a shared understanding about diagnosis, prognosis and treatment (Poole and Higgo, 2006; Priebe *et al.*, 2005).

Effective communication skills in mental health consultation makes interactions less stressful for all parties and is associated with increased patient satisfaction and the possibility of better adherence to treatment (McCabe *et al.*, 2002).

COMMUNICATION SKILLS TRAINING FOR MENTAL HEALTH PROFESSIONALS

A definition of communication skills training in mental health is any form of structured didactic, e-learning and experiential (e.g. role playing) training targeted at mental health professionals in order to develop proficiency in effective mental health consultations with patients (Kurtz *et al.*, 2005).

Recent communication skills teaching to medical undergraduates utilises a variety of models. Examples of these are the 'three-function model' (Cole and Bird, 2000) and the Calgary–Cambridge model (Kurtz *et al.*, 2005).

These models divide the mental health consultation into a number of tasks:
➤ introductions
➤ information gathering
➤ explanation and planning
➤ closing the consultation.

In order for the mental health professional to achieve the above tasks, they will have to follow such processes as building a patient-centred relationship and structuring the consultation.

To carry out these tasks and processes successfully, the clinician has to use a number of skills:

➤ active listening
➤ using open and closed questions
➤ summarising
➤ signposting, chunking and checking
➤ recognising, acknowledging and validating patients' ideas
➤ eliciting patients' concerns and expectations.

In this book, we will use the Calgary–Cambridge model (Kurtz *et al.*, 2005; Silverman *et al.*, 2005).

In more recent years, attempts have been made to incorporate brief, succinct and comprehensive skills from other training approaches such as motivational interviewing and cognitive behavioural therapy into psychiatric consultations in order to improve concordance with antipsychotic medication, insight into illness and change of attitudes to treatment (Rollnick *et al.*, 2008; Barrowclough *et al.*, 2010).

The training of undergraduate and graduate students requires the use of experiential learning methods, for example role play involving detailed scenarios of patients with severe mental health conditions. The part of the patient is best played by an experienced simulated patient. The trainees practice the skills in role plays in groups or in one-to-one sessions and receive individual feedback on their performance from the consultation skills tutor. Visual recording is useful for later review by the tutor and student and for the student to take away from the session. According to Silverman *et al.* (2005), experiential learning is the best method of learning and retaining communication skills and is supported by the majority of evidence in this area.

Within the last 10 years a number of e-learning resources have become available as an aid to developing communication skills. These include model consultations which can reinforce trainees' learning (http://webcampus.drexelmed.edu/doccom/user), although no good measure yet exists of the effectiveness of this technique compared to experiential training.

Overall, there is little evidence linking communication skills training of mental health professionals with treatment outcomes (Hassan *et al.*, 2007). With the introduction of such training in undergraduate and postgraduate medical education and psychiatric settings, the next decades will hopefully produce more evidence in this area. In summary, the few studies that exist suggest that shared decision-making interventions for people with mental health conditions do not prolong the mental health consultation (Duncan *et al.*, 2010) and the competent use of communication skills during the session does predict improvement of symptoms in depression (Hassan *et al.*, 2007).

Future studies are needed to continue the improvement of the training of mental health professionals, the education of patients and primary care professionals, and professionals in other treatment settings to achieve best outcomes for patients.

In this book we will address not only the core aspects of the psychiatric consultation but also some more specific areas, such as working with families and young people, dealing with emotions, breaking bad news and mental health consultations in primary care.

As with the general mental health consultation, research in the above areas is also quite sparse.

For example, a recent American study looked at what aspects of mental health communication skills training predict parent and child outcomes in paediatric primary care (Wissow *et al.*, 2011). This small randomised controlled trial trained 31 clinicians with a mean of 15.6 years working experience and backgrounds in paediatrics or family practice to use communication skills in time management, problem solving, managing anger, agenda setting, problem formulation, advice giving and managing resistance.

An interesting finding of this study is that trained clinicians showed an increase in patient-centredness (e.g. eliciting patients' ideas, concerns, expectations, feelings, thoughts and developing an understanding of the effects the illness has had on their lives). This study also revealed that clinicians who had received the training used it preferentially and retained certain skills but not others. These were: setting the agenda, managing anger and managing time. The authors suggest that extending training time may not be the solution to learning all the communication skills necessary to carry out efficient and effective consultations, but that changing the way trainees receive feedback may be the way forward. For example, observing or videotaping trainees' real-life consultations and giving them immediate feedback would be impacting but resource-intensive (Wissow *et al.*, 2011).

In the UK over the past few decades, primary care settings have embraced communication skills training more eagerly than other medical specialties. A large part of the prevention, identification and management of mental health problems also takes place in primary care settings. A Cochrane review on interventions for providers to promote a patient-centred approach in clinical consultations identified a number of studies carried out in primary care settings (Lewin *et al.*, 2007). The reviewed studies recruited patients with physical conditions, chronic conditions (e.g. diabetes) and patients with psychosocial problems. This review provides a good insight on the effectiveness of communication skills training, and as with the previous studies it suggests the need for more refined and bigger-scale studies. The authors (Lewin *et al.*, 2007) conclude that communication skills training increases patient-centredness when this is measured in terms of the skills used to clarify patients' concerns and beliefs, discussion of treatment options and empathising with the patient. They also suggest that most studies on communication skills interventions used a variety of non-direct measures of patient-centredness, which means there is no gold standard measure for patient-centredness to date. This review provides some evidence that training health care professionals to use patient-centred skills does improve patients' satisfaction with their care.

A lot of communication skills textbooks devote substantial sections to dealing with emotions. We will do the same with a specific focus on patients with mental health problems. Again, there is very little research on this topic. A fairly recent qualitative study looked at the experiences of patients with schizophrenia in relation to grief (Mauritz and van Meijel, 2009). Using in-depth interviews and excluding patients with clinical depression, the authors explored patients' feelings of loss and ways of coping. Participants experienced both internal (e.g. not belonging, isolated) and external (e.g. grief, sombreness, desperation, guilt, anger) feelings of loss and went through an intense period of grief before they came to terms with their illness. Knowledge and understanding of their condition, identification with other patients with the same condition and searching for meaning were among the coping mechanisms they employed. This piece of research suggests that patients with severe, chronic mental health conditions go through the same grief processes as people with chronic physical conditions (Kubler-Ross, 1997). Research evidence in this area will help to put in place mechanisms to help patients cope with their grief and reduce mortality rates.

THE WAY FORWARD

The challenge of research in this area is to quantify the effects of communication skills interventions on health status. As a consequence, it makes it difficult to generate funding and promote training in health-care systems with many competing demands for research, training and development. Future research needs to refine both the communication skills training interventions and the method of quantifying impact.

It needs to answer the questions:

➤ What are the best teaching methods of communication skills training?
➤ How intense should they be?
➤ How long should the learning last?
➤ How do the behaviours and attitudes of the mental health professionals change because of this training?
➤ What is the impact of the skills learnt on patients' behaviour and health status outcomes?
➤ Does such training change the culture of an organisation and how care is delivered?
➤ Does it produce more satisfied mental health care professionals and patients?

As the authors of the included studies suggest, communication skills training for mental health professionals and its impact on patient outcomes is in its infancy. We still have more questions than answers in this field. However, the small research evidence base that exists provides a stepping stone for expansion and exciting future opportunities.

REFERENCES

Barrowclough C, Haddock G, Wykes T, *et al.* Integrated motivational interviewing and cognitive behavioural therapy for people with psychosis and comorbid substance misuse: a randomised controlled trial. *BMJ.* 2010; **341**: c6325.

Cole SA, Bird J. *The Medical Interview: the three-function approach.* 2nd ed. St Louis, MO: Mosby; 2000.

Duncan E, Best C, Hagen S. Shared decision making interventions for people with mental health conditions. *Cochrane Database Syst Rev.* 2010; **1**: CD007297.

Harris EC, Barraclough B. Excess mortality of mental disorder. *Brit J Psychiat.* 1998; **173**: 11–53.

Hassan I, McCabe R, Priebe S. Professional-patient communication in the treatment of mental illness: a review. *Commun Med.* 2007; **4**(2): 141–52.

Jenkins R, Bebbington P, Brugha T, *et al.* British Psychiatric Morbidity Survey. *Int Rev Psychiatr.* 2003; **15**: 14–18.

Kubler-Ross E. *On Death and Dying.* New York, NY: Touchstone; 1997.

Kurtz S, Silverman J, Draper J. *Teaching and Learning Communication Skills in Medicine.* 2nd ed. Oxford: Radcliffe; 2005.

Lewin SA, Skea ZC, Entwistle V, *et al.* Interventions for providers to promote a patient-centred approach in clinical consultations. *Cochrane Database Syst Rev.* 2007; **4**: CD000409.

Mauritz M, van Meijel B. Loss and grief in patients with schizophrenia: on living in another world. *Arch Psychiatr Nurs.* 2009; **23**(3): 251–60.

McCabe R, Heath C, Burns T, *et al.* Engagement of patients with psychosis in the medical consultation: a conversation analytic study. *BMJ.* 2002; **325**: 1148–51.

Murray C, Lopez A. *The Global Burden of Disease.* Harvard, CT: Harvard University Press; 1996.

Poole R, Higgo R. *Psychiatric Interviewing and Assessment.* Cambridge: Cambridge University Press; 2006.

Priebe S, Watts J, Chase M, *et al.* Processes of disengagement and engagement in assertive outreach patients: qualitative study. *Brit J Psychiat.* 2005; **187**: 438–43.

Rollnick S, Miller WR, Butler CC. *Motivational Interviewing in Health Care.* London: Guildford; 2008.

Silverman J, Kurtz S, Draper J. *Skills for Communicating with Patients.* 2nd ed. Oxford: Radcliffe; 2005.

Singleton N, Bumpstead R, O'Brien M, *et al.* Psychiatric morbidity among adults living in private households, 2000. *Int Rev Psychiatr.* 2003; **15**: 65–73.

Wissow L, Gadomski A, Roter D, *et al.* Aspects of mental health communication skills training that predict parent and child outcomes in paediatric primary care. *Patient Educ Couns.* 2011; **82**(2): 226–32.

CHAPTER 2

Taking a good psychiatric history

Jonathan Wilson

LEARNING OUTCOMES

- To understand the elements of a full psychiatric history and mental state examination
- To understand how to structure a mental state examination
- To understand how the history informs the management and treatment plan
- To consider how to approach patients with mental illness and sensitively collect and formulate information using applied Calgary–Cambridge techniques

THE PURPOSE OF THE PSYCHIATRIC HISTORY

The ultimate goal of a psychiatric intervention is to elicit sufficient information from a patient in order to allow a considered diagnosis (or a range of diagnoses) to be made and then to discuss the treatment options available. In this respect, the psychiatric history does not differ from standard medical or surgical histories. The main difference is in the range of information often needed to produce a robust opinion to share with the patient.

Psychiatric practice has evolved over many years. Its origins lie in neurology, to which, thanks to the insights of Freud and the psychoanalysts, layers of complexity were added. Over many years, our conceptual understanding of psychiatric 'illness' has shifted, often shaped by prevailing social pressures. Diagnoses come and go, as does society's willingness to see people as 'ill' rather than their difficulties stemming from a social origin. Previous diagnostic categories such as homosexuality and addiction are continually being reframed as quickly as new diagnoses have evolved (e.g. social phobia, Asperger's syndrome or attention deficit hyperactivity disorder). Our understanding of the significance and validity of certain assumed prodromal syndromes such as schizotypal personality disorder remains unclear. Indeed, many of our diagnostic classifications are accepted as having poor inter-rater reliability, yet we continue to use them. Examples of these might be personality disorders or milder forms of depressive disorders.

Despite this, if psychiatry is to provide evidenced-based and standardised interventions, we need a common understanding from which to work. Indeed, this uncertainty is, for many, the attraction of psychiatry. At one level we are dealing with what makes each individual unique; our personal experience, genetic make-up, specific life events, etc., and trying to offer shared understanding and assistance.

Over the last few decades, diagnoses have often driven the funding and treatment packages an individual receives. However, at various times, it has been noted that diagnostic patterns for, say, bipolar affective disorder and schizophrenia, have differed substantially between various countries. Every culture has its own subtle or overt understanding of what constitutes mental health and mental illness, differing levels of social support, and different types of traumatic experiences which might affect an individual's development and shape their resilience and view of the world. A robust and useful psychiatric history needs to balance all of these factors and yet still arrive at something meaningful both to the patient and the wider medical or professional body. This balancing act requires a sophisticated degree of background knowledge, applied in a sensitive way so that a comprehensive shared understanding can be achieved. It should encapsulate psychotherapeutic understanding, yet balance this with more biological theoretical frameworks. No mean feat!

THE PSYCHIATRIC HISTORY COMPARED WITH A MEDICAL HISTORY

In psychiatry, as in all medical specialities, diagnosis is made on the basis of history, examination and investigations. What constitutes a good psychiatric history is, in many ways, hardly different from a standard medical history. Of course, the emphasis may differ, as may the weight given to symptoms and signs. There are few clear physical signs to support our diagnoses. Whilst every patient should have a physical examination in order to exclude an organic cause for their presentation, the *Mental State Examination* is the nearest that psychiatrists can get to objective, reproducible evidence which might support one diagnosis over another. This will be discussed in more detail later in this chapter.

In the main, though, the 'evidence' needed to arrive at a diagnosis is no different from usual medical practice. The order of the headings varies slightly between authors, but invariably the content is the same as that shown in Table 2.1:

TABLE 2.1 The psychiatric history

- Demographic information (age, marital status, referral information, race, etc.)
- Presenting or chief complaint (as the patient sees it)
- History of presenting complaint (including history of an informant where appropriate)
- Previous psychiatric history (including details of each 'illness' episode)
- Previous medical history – past and present
- Current medication or drug history (including adherence)
- Family history
- Social history
- Personal history
- Premorbid personality
- Drug and alcohol history
- Forensic history
- Mental State Examination
- Formulation and summary
- Differential diagnosis
- Physical examination
- Risk assessment
- Treatment plan

It will be apparent that this structure is identical to general medical histories. What is different, however, is the depth of information required in order to arrive at a formulation and diagnosis. A fuller guide to what might be included in a psychiatric history can be found in Appendix 2 at the end of the book.

Diagnoses in psychiatry are generally made according to standard (and slowly changing) internationally recognised criteria. In the UK and much of the rest of the world, we use the International Classification of Mental and Behavioural Disorders, 10th edition (ICD-10), although an alternative, largely American system is also common – the Diagnostic and Statistical Manual, version 4 (DSM-IV). These systems are similar, and each has clear criteria upon which to base one's diagnostic opinions (Castle *et al.*, 2006; First *et al.*, 1996).

When initially starting out in psychiatry, and indeed as a general rule of good practice, clinicians should note that taking a thorough history is essential. At the outset of a consultation, it is difficult to know which areas will be of importance (e.g. recent medical events, genetic predisposition, childhood trauma, substance use). Often a complex interaction of many factors will be present. Only once all of the information has been gathered can it be synthesised to arrive at an educated hypothesis as to the totality of what might lie behind a person's difficulties – a formulation. It is reasonable in all psychiatric consultations to ask the question: *Why is this person presenting at this point in time with these particular difficulties?*

This leads to further questions relevant to why a person has presented – what features have predisposed, precipitated and perpetuated the situation. These can be simplified to a series of domains using the 'bio-psycho-social model' of psychiatry (Table 2.2):

TABLE 2.2 The bio-psycho-social model of psychiatry

	Biological factors	*Psychological factors*	*Social factors*
Predisposing factors	e.g. Family history of bipolar disorder	e.g. Avoidant coping style	e.g. Multiple schools and peer groups in childhood
Precipitating factors	e.g. Cocaine use	e.g. Relationship breakup	e.g. Loss of job
Perpetuating factors	e.g. Lack of acceptance of role of medication	e.g. Avoidant coping style, poor self-esteem	e.g. Housing difficulties

The example in Table 2.2 above is clearly an oversimplification but illustrates the complexity of why a person is presenting and what might have led to this situation, and begins to hint at which areas might need to be addressed in order to help someone overcome their difficulties. This formulation will be unique and relevant to a patient and should be arrived at collaboratively. Simply telling a person that they have bipolar affective disorder and suggesting a tablet will clearly not be sufficient!

GATHERING A PSYCHIATRIC HISTORY

All too often, busy clinicians forget that taking a history is in itself a therapeutic experience, the aim of which is to encourage the patient to explain anything potentially relevant and then work with the clinician on devising an agreed formulation, possible diagnosis and treatment plan. Arguably, if one presents with a specific pain or physical ailment, then shortcuts can be taken. Whilst not ideal, under these circumstances the overt agenda is easier to agree on and the depth of information required will be less in some areas. In such instances, screening questions may quickly guide both the clinician and patient to a reasonable conclusion.

Unfortunately, in psychiatry, matters are usually not so straightforward. As a rule, patients are anxious, fearful, ashamed – a whole range of initial expectations. Each of these may interfere with the interview process. Merely firing questions at someone is unlikely to yield good information, and so the whole process is likely to be flawed. Inevitably, this leads to poor or incomplete treatment plans. At worst, it is likely to discourage the patient and the therapeutic aspects of feeling listened to, understood and seeing a way forward will be lost. Excellent consultation skills and communication skills are essential.

There is a need to find out specific information and ask about a variety of domains in a person's life. Merely asking about an issue (e.g. *'Do you have a house?'*) is almost pointless. It is the quality of the information gathered, the awareness of the impact on a person's life and the meaning attached to an issue or event which guides treatment. Balancing a patient's agenda, ideas, concerns and expectations with the clinician's is a tricky but skilful task. Done well, it flows like a guided conversation; done badly, it is stilted and jars.

It is also true that specific, technical information is necessary to inform which questions to ask. If a patient has seemingly irrational fears, then focusing on a line of questions to clarify certain themes will be necessary at some point. However, if the clinician is not familiar with psychotic disorders, then it will be difficult to achieve. Nevertheless, trying to order a patient's story allows a senior colleague to begin to understand the issue to hand.

ELICITING A PSYCHIATRIC HISTORY

Any decent interview starts even before the patient is seen. The setting needs to be right. Who would want to speak to a stranger in detail about their life in a corridor or busy ward? A safe, comfortable space, free from interruptions, including telephone calls, is a necessity. Be mindful of safety issues and ensure that you have checked that it is suitable to interview someone, that if necessary others know where you are and how long you will be and that the room is suitable. If there are any issues of risk to yourself, ensure that you are seated with unimpeded access to the door or that you are in an appropriately equipped room with outward opening doors. If in an acute inpatient setting, make sure that you are carrying a personal alarm with which to summon assistance if necessary. Whilst this sounds dramatic, if you prepare and plan properly, then only very rarely should it be necessary to terminate an interview or summon help.

Consider the referral information:

➤ What does it tell you?
➤ What issues immediately stand out?
➤ What concerns and expectations might the patient have?
➤ What other information can you establish?
➤ Are there any areas which you might need to ensure that you cover?
➤ Are there some existing medical notes, and if so, what do they tell you about what has been tried before and the likely direction the consultation might go?
➤ Is there a need to ensure that your consultation is different?
➤ How would you achieve that?

Initiating a consultation

Where your consultation might lead is covered throughout the rest of this book. The principles remain the same, however: you are trying to conduct a therapeutic interaction designed to achieve a shared understanding of the nature of the problems and how they might be treated. You may possess special experience of treating psychological problems which you need to bring into the consultation. However, the more you can agree a collaborative formulation and treatment plan, the better the outcome is likely to be. There are special situations which require special skills – e.g. an angry patient, a deluded patient – but even here your aims are largely the same.

The Calgary–Cambridge model provides an excellent framework upon which to base most aspects of your consultation. They are most definitely skills which can be honed and individualised and they do require practice and active feedback about performance. The model breaks down the opening stages of a consultation as below:

Getting started

Establishing initial rapport
Greets patient and obtains patient's name
Introduces self, role and nature of interview; obtains consent if necessary
Demonstrates respect and interest, attends to patient's physical comfort

Identifying the reason(s) for the consultation
Identifies **the patient's problems or the issues that the patient wishes to address with appropriate** opening question (e.g. *What problems brought you to see the GP?* or *What would you like to discuss today?*)
Listens attentively to the patient's opening statement, without interrupting or directing patient's response
Confirms list and screens for further problems (e.g. *So that's headaches and tiredness; anything else . . .?*)
Negotiates agenda taking both patient's and clinician's needs into account

These sound like obvious and straightforward stages. However, all too often the interview falls down at this initial step. Bearing in mind that we tend to decide our attitude to a stranger within the first few seconds of meeting them, the opening remarks and discussion are critical. Patients come with expectations – not always positive. Your task is to understand these: ideally, use these to inform you about their underlying psychological processes and procedures and use this to elicit even more information about why this person is presenting at this point in time and what is maintaining the situation.

Start by showing interest in the person. Orientate your conversation in the 'real world'. Explain what your role is and what is going to happen. Make it clear that you are there to help understand what is going on. Clarify any points which you do not understand. Model inquisitiveness and understanding. Overtly make it clear that you can empathise and realise that certain themes might be uncomfortable. Try to remain open-minded and neutral. Thus:

> Clinician: *Hello Mrs Wright. My name is _____ . I am one of the* (psychiatrists/clinicians/nurses, etc.) *who works with the mental health team. Your GP has asked that we meet in order to try to understand in a little more detail what has been happening of late. Please take a seat . . .* (shake hands).
>
> Mrs Wright: *Yes, of course.*
>
> Clinician: *Was that your husband waiting outside? If you'd like him to join us, that is perfectly all right with me. In fact he might be able to help us get a better understanding of what has been going on lately.*
>
> Mrs Wright: *No thank you – I'd prefer to talk to you on my own. Perhaps he could join us later?*
>
> Clinician: *That's a good idea. Are you comfortable; it's a hot day, would you like a glass of water?*
>
> Mrs Wright: *No thank you – I'm fine. Just feeling a little nervous.*
>
> Clinician: *Well, there is really no need to be nervous. If you'd like to stop talking for a while at any point, just let me know. I had hoped that we could talk for around 45 minutes and hopefully try to work out what has been happening and when. Everything we say will be confidential although we do share information within the team and with your GP if you are agreeable. By the end of our meeting hopefully we will be able to agree if we can be of any help and if so what might happen next. Could we start with what you think might be the main issues?*

There are many ways to begin to talk with someone. Remember that explaining about your life to a stranger is a novel experience for most people and actively building up trust is an absolute necessity. Each opening to an interview needs to be tailored to an individual's needs; some people may need a longer 'safe' preamble in order to feel secure; others may prefer to get straight to the point. Asking general information usually helps this process (*Did you find the building all right?*; *Did you manage to park okay?*, etc.). However, if you persist with these questions, they can seem clumsy or irritating. They do show interest in a person rather than a problem, though, and can help the session flow more naturally.

From the outset of a consultation, you will be noting their behaviour, clothing, how they relate to you, whether they are distracted, how relaxed they are, how their mood seems, whether their thoughts flow smoothly, etc. This is information which you will need to remember and use to guide your consultation as you begin to focus in on key aspects as the interview progresses.

Pay particular attention to the patient's opening description of their problems. In my experience, this can yield a tremendous amount of information and be a powerful tool in forming a collaborative relationship. Let the patient speak at length if necessary. Facilitate them continuing to speak with body language, your facial expression and invitations to continue. Give the patient every opportunity to describe their perception of the nature of their problems. Meanwhile, listen both to what they are saying and how they are saying it. Does speaking about their difficulties provoke emotion or anxiety? Do they need to minimise or avoid thinking about their problems? Do they as yet have a clear understanding of what might be happening and why? Do they think that they are unwell? If not, what do they think might be wrong?

This opening section of the consultation should serve to guide the next part of the interview. Start to clarify certain points – perhaps offer a brief summary of what the person has said. Remember that you are trying to form a collaborative therapeutic relationship with the patient and to model your role in the interview – that of someone who is interested. This opening section may take a few minutes but generally this is time well spent. It leads on to setting an agenda so that you are both clear about the parameters of the session, i.e.:

> Clinician: *Thank you. You have just told me about what might have been going wrong for you over the last few months* (summarise?). *What I'd like to suggest is that we now look in a little more detail at certain aspects of this and at your life in general to see if we can reach an understanding about why all of this is happening and what we can do to help. We have about 40 minutes to speak about these things and perhaps, if that isn't enough time, we can meet again? Before we start, I wonder if you have any things which you would particularly like to talk about?*

This raises the concept of ICE – Ideas, Concerns, Expectations – an undervalued tool in conducting a successful consultation. By explicitly addressing any fear or ICE an individual has, useful information can be fed into the formulation and any potential barriers to conducting a successful interview can be addressed.

Gathering information

The interview now moves into a phase of gathering information about the nature, potential causes and onset of the patient's difficulties. Again, the Calgary–Cambridge model provides an excellent guide to progressing the interview. By demonstrating a willingness to understand the detail of how a problem developed, what led up to it, what help has been offered to date and what effect it has had and the impact of the problem on the patient's wider life, you can begin to piece together with a patient how their difficulties have evolved. Often it can help to structure the interview along the way and at each stage, clarify the information gathered and summarise before moving on in order to ensure that you have appreciated things correctly. For example:

> Clinician: *If I'm correct you have spoken about three main issues – the problems in your relationship, the death of your father and feeling increasingly depressed over the last 6 months. I wonder if we could spend a bit of time looking at each of these in a little more detail?*

The interview would then move on to explore the reason for the consultation in more detail.

Exploration of patient's problems

Encourages patient to tell the story of the problem(s) from when first started to the present in own words (clarifying reason for presenting now)

Uses open and closed questioning technique, appropriately moving from open to closed

Listens attentively, allowing patient to complete statements without interruption and leaving space for patient to think before answering or go on after pausing

Facilitates patient's responses verbally and non-verbally, e.g. use of encouragement, silence, repetition, paraphrasing, interpretation

Picks up verbal and non-verbal **cues** (body language, speech, facial expression, affect); checks out and acknowledges as appropriate

Clarifies patient's statements that are unclear or need amplification (e.g. *'Could you explain what you mean by light headed'*)

Periodically summarises to verify own understanding of what the patient has said; invites patient to correct interpretation or provide further information

Uses concise, **easily understood questions and comments**, avoids or adequately explains jargon

Establishes dates and sequence of events

Actively **determines and appropriately explores**:

- patient's **ideas** (i.e. beliefs re cause)
- patient's **concerns** (i.e. worries) regarding each problem
- patient's **expectations** (i.e. goals, what help the patient had expected for each problem)
- effects: how each problem **affects** the patient's life

Encourages patient to express feelings

As the interview progresses, you will at times need explicitly to move on to other areas within the psychiatric history headings – summarising each time before doing so and signposting where you are going next. Many times, however, the interview may flow better as a conversation in which you fill in your 'blank' on the history pro forma and only signpost on occasion when moving to cover a specific area. For each area you will need to be clear that you have sufficient information. For example, when eliciting a drug and alcohol history, if your initial screening questions suggest that there may be some issues, then you will need to be as specific as possible about drug use, amounts taken, routes of administration, the time course of substance use, etc.

THE MENTAL STATE EXAMINATION

The Mental State Examination is psychiatry's attempt to describe objectively the patient's current state of mind. By convention, this description is arbitrarily broken down into a series of subsections which follow in a standard order. There is some minor variation in this order, but the headings remain the same. These headings are shown in Table 2.3 below.

The Mental State Examination (MSE) stems from the pioneering work of Karl Jaspers, who described psychopathology, which is further broken down into explanatory and descriptive phenomenology. There are two distinct parts to descriptive psychopathology – the observation of behaviour and the assessment of subjective experiences. Each of these elements is contained within the MSE. In order to describe accurately the patient's subjective experiences, one must use empathy (i.e. arriving at a shared empathic understanding of what a patient is experiencing in order to accurately discern the exact nature of the subjective experience). Whilst describing internal experiences in this way is not truly objective, it does provide a relatively reliable method of ensuring that each assessment of a person's mental state uses the same criteria to define a symptom or experience.

TABLE 2.3 The Mental State Examination

- Appearance
- Behaviour
- Speech
- Mood and affect
- Thought processes
    - form
    - content
- Perceptions
- Cognition
- Insight

Patients' distress can be classified in a variety of ways. Most common is to categorise these experiences such that they eventually cluster into a recognisable syndrome, such as 'depression' or 'anxiety'. There is considerable overlap between many diagnostic groups (people with psychosis often feel anxious, people with anorexia often have fixed beliefs about their body image); however, rigorously applied, these categories are a useful concept to allow communication and research and development of the psychiatric practice. Standardised semi-structured questionnaires such as the Structured Clinical Interview for DSM-IV (SCID) can be used as a means of exploring a patient's mental state (First *et al.*, 1996). It should be noted that in clinical practice, the MSE is completed during or alongside the interview, not added on at the end as a specific procedure. By the end of the interview, it may be necessary to ask screening questions or to clarify specific points, however.

THE DOMAINS OF THE MENTAL STATE EXAMINATION
Appearance
In daily life as well as in clinical practice, our starting point for any assessment is observing the person in front of us. In psychiatry, any number of observations about a person's appearance can give useful clues as to their inner psychological world. Excessively brightly coloured or bizarre clothing may suggest mania. Their degree of self-care, their weight, height, tattoos or piercings may each suggest (but are *not* diagnostic of) a person's attitudes, beliefs or lifestyle. Significant self-neglect, malnutrition, nicotine-stained fingers, poor dental care, etc. again all help suggest likely internal psychological states.

Behaviour
Can the person sit still? Are they moving too quickly – speeded up – or are they slowed down? Do they fidget, are they distracted by possibly external stimuli which only they can hear, are there any unusual behaviours? There are many aspects of a person's behaviour which, put together with the history and mental state examination, may help confirm or give evidence which points towards a certain diagnosis or syndrome.

Speech
A patient's speech is assessed by observing their spontaneous speech and describing this. Commonly, it is assessed in terms of rate, rhythm, tone and volume, articulation, choice of words (made up words – neologisms), echolalia (repetition of the patient's own words) and many other aspects. Each lends evidence towards an internal process – whether functional (i.e. psychological in origin) or biological/organic (e.g. a stroke or dementing illness). This domain addresses the *production* of speech and mechanics rather than the content, which is more linked to thought content and thought form.

Mood and affect

Often it is difficult to differentiate between mood and affect. There are many definitions which have all often been used interchangeably. Oyebode (2008), in his excellent book on descriptive psychopathology, describes *affect* as being used to describe differentiated specific feelings towards objects, whilst *mood* is a more prolonged prevailing state or disposition. That is to say, affect is what we observe by facial expression, reactions, etc. which are both deliberately and unintentionally conveyed, whilst a mood state describes the underlying state of mind. Affect has been likened to the waves on the sea, whilst mood is more akin to the underlying tidal flows.

Any description of mood and affect includes both what the observer sees and the patient's subjective description of their feelings plus somatic or biological features which are more pervasive. Affect may be blunted (in schizophrenia), restricted (in depression), incongruous (i.e. out of keeping with the topic or emotion of the topic being discussed), or heightened (in mania). Affect provides valuable information about a patient's internal state of mind and how this is manifest. An assessment of mood traditionally contains a description of the patient's feelings, attitudes towards themselves (worthlessness, hopelessness) or their attitudes towards the world around them (negative, overly positive, etc.).

Importantly, this section of the MSE also needs to cover in detail any thoughts, plans, intent or actions a patient may have related with regard to deliberate self-harm or suicide.

Thought processes

Disturbances of thought are traditionally subdivided into disturbances of the form of thinking and disturbances of the content.

Disturbances of the form or flow of thinking occur in many conditions. Thinking may be slowed (retardation), lacking substance (poverty of thought), increased in rate (typically associated with mania). There may be perseveration (i.e. a pattern where a person keeps returning to a limited series of ideas). Thoughts may be interrupted or disorganised. The associations between one thought and the next can be altered in a number of ways (e.g. in schizophrenia, the classically described disturbance of thought form is that of loosened associations between one thought and the next, also known as 'knight's move thinking' since the first thought has no logical connection to the next). In mania, the disturbance of thought form is typically an acceleration of the flow of thoughts with some logical association between them but often very tenuous. This is known as 'flight of ideas' and, in its extreme form, the association can simply be that words rhyme – a state known as 'punning'. There are many other descriptive terms to describe disturbed thought form, such as circumstantial thinking, derailment, fusion, thought blocking, etc.

Thought content describes what the patient is thinking. These may be 'normal' thoughts (i.e. not demonstrating any abnormalities) or may have varying degrees of preoccupations. What constitutes a normal content may vary depending upon the setting or the cultural and social system within which the patient lives.

The content will become apparent with careful questioning, listening and clarification, throughout the interview. Any abnormalities should be clear if open-ended questions are used with further clarifications. The intensity, associated emotion, extent to which thoughts are considered one's own and whether the patient can accept any unusual thoughts as being in some way unreasonable or unwanted are all important factors to consider.

Preoccupations, worries, obsessions (an unpleasant, unwanted, intrusive thought that cannot be suppressed), phobias (an irrational dread of an object or situation that does not pose any threat), overvalued ideas (a false belief held with conviction but not with delusional intensity), and delusions (a fixed usually false belief which is out of keeping with the patient's educational, cultural and social background held with extraordinary conviction and subjective certainty) may be present. It is very important to clarify as far as possible the exact nature of these abnormalities as they have great diagnostic significance.

Perceptions

The mechanisms by which we perceive the world can be distorted in any sensory modality. Broadly speaking, there are two main types of sensory disturbance. Illusions are false sensory perceptions in the presence of a real external stimulus (e.g. a coat hanging behind a door being misperceived as a person). A true hallucination is a perception without a percept (i.e. there is no external stimulus).

Hallucinations and perceptual disturbances can occur in any of the five senses, although auditory and visual are the most common. They can occur in many organic (biological/physical illnesses) conditions and need not purely be functional (part of a major mental illness) in origin. As can be imagined, there are many types of specific perceptual disturbances which are often underpinned by delusional beliefs. Many of these technical terms are associated with specific conditions, e.g. hearing one's thoughts spoken out loud (Oyebode, 2008).

Assessing psychotic beliefs and experiences is a complicated procedure – if an experience is perceived as real, then how can it be discussed with an 'as if' quality? These complicated areas are covered elsewhere in this book. Specific tools can offer invaluable help in providing prompts and clarity with one's line of questioning. The diagnostic interview for psychosis is one such tool which can help in everyday practice. This is described further in Chapter 5.

Cognition

This section of the Mental State Examination concerns itself with core organic brain functions. It includes assessment of alertness, orientation, attention, memory, the mechanics of speech and language (e.g. dysarthria), visuospatial functioning and frontal-executive abilites. For many patients, a gross assessment of this will have taken place throughout the interview. For some patients, specific testing may be indicated (e.g. the Mini-Mental State Examination or a similar global assessment test of cognitive functioning). For a small minority of patients, further specialist testing may be required (e.g. IQ testing or similar).

Obviously, any degree of psychological distress will impair performance in a number of areas. Severe psychological conditions (e.g. severe obsessive-compulsive disorder or florid psychosis) may significantly impair gross or specific cognitive testing, and allowance needs to be made for this. Cognitive assessment is discussed in more detail in Chapter 8.

Insight

To have insight into the nature of one's difficulties requires a number of factors; accepting that there is a problem, recognising that treatment or changes may be necessary and an ability to recognise that certain difficulties or experiences are abnormal or pathological. In practice, many patients may disagree or have a different (but potentially or partially acceptable) alternative explanation. Thus a description of insight should not merely be 'present' or 'absent'. Rather, it should describe the patient's understanding of their condition and acceptance to seek or comply with help as compared to the clinician's. Both opinions are potentially equally valid, and this section allows the patient's understanding of what is needed to be made manifest.

Conclusion

The art and science of psychiatric history taking is a complex one. As can be seen, it requires background theoretical knowledge (in order to know which questions to ask), but needs to be conducted in a manner which facilitates engagement and exploration. Done well, it is undoubtedly therapeutic in itself. It should culminate with a clear shared understanding of why certain issues are presenting at this point in time and identify what needs to be addressed to resolve matters. The remaining chapters in this book are aimed at assisting clinicians in achieving this task and, if necessary, being able to demonstrate this to examiners.

REFERENCES

Castle D, Jablensky A, McGrath J, *et al*. The Diagnostic Interview for Psychoses (DIP): development, reliability and applications. *Psychol Med*. 2006; **36**: 69–80.

First M, Spitzer R, Gibbon M, *et al*. *Structured Clinical Interview for DSM-IV for Axis I Disorders (SCID-I/P) (Version 2.0)*. New York, NY: New York State Psychiatric Institute; 1996.

Oyebode F. *Sims' Symptoms in the Mind: an introduction to descriptive psychopathology*. Edinburgh: Saunders Elsevier; 2008.

CHAPTER 3

Mental health assessment of anxiety and depression

Nick Viale and Rebecca Horne

LEARNING OUTCOMES

- To use the Calgary–Cambridge skills associated with information gathering from a patient with anxiety and depression
- To utilise the appropriate skills for taking a history from a patient with anxiety and depression
- To describe the aspects of appearance, behaviour and mood of the Mental State Examination in relation to a patient with anxiety and depression

INTRODUCTION

Depression and anxiety are frequently occurring psychiatric disorders which can easily be missed in medical practice. Accurate recognition and diagnosis is very dependent on the skills of the clinician. In this session we will focus on the assessment of a patient with depression, but will highlight the differences between this presentation and that of a patient with an anxiety disorder.

Interviewing patients with mental illness highlights the importance of the core Calgary–Cambridge skills of gathering information, in particular of taking an accurate clinical history, and building a therapeutic relationship with the patient.

DEPRESSION

A patient attending with physical symptoms may have a comorbid psychiatric illness or somatic symptoms of an underlying depression, which are perceived as a physical illness. An accurate diagnosis depends on the skill of the clinician in taking a history and conducting the Mental State Examination, in combination with Calgary–Cambridge skills. The Calgary–Cambridge process skills help the patient to tell their story – as well as assisting the clinician to learn about their ideas, concerns and expectations.

Many depressed patients feel that they do not deserve to take up their clinician's time and, as part of their illness, feel that it is not possible for the clinician to listen sympathetically and understand them. As a consequence, they may feel that they receive less helpful care than they need and deserve.

A focus on building the relationship right from the start of the consultation will encourage the patient to 'open up', to share feelings, to tell the story in their own words and to develop a working therapeutic rapport. Expressing empathy, providing support and asking difficult questions sensitively will help the clinician to elicit key facts, such as whether the depressed patient has a severe and sustained disturbance of mood, accompanying feelings of worthlessness, loss of interest and morbid guilt as well as alterations in energy levels, concentration, appetite, weight and sleep pattern.

It is paramount to discover the level of a patient's depression and whether they have suicidal ideation, with thoughts of hopelessness, self-harm or suicide (covered in greater detail in Chapter 4, Assessing Risk to Self). These aspects will influence negotiating a management plan later in a consultation.

Employment of open questions and precision in using closed questions are important and should be combined with a compassionate approach and the willingness to witness what the patient is experiencing. Patients who are very depressed may respond well to open questions and empathic statements, which may help them to express more readily their feelings and reveal further information. Others may need the clinician to use a series of closed and directed questions to help them tell a story, parts of which, such as details of suicidal intent, may be difficult for them to disclose. The clinician has to make a judgement on how long to persevere with trying to 'open up' a severely depressed patient, in an attempt to build rapport and obtain the information required, or when to move to more closed questions to elucidate how depressed the patient is, how likely they are to attempt suicide and whether it is safe to allow the patient home.

The clinician, in witnessing what the patient is experiencing, may himself experience a variety of emotions felt by the patient, including sadness, desperation, hopelessness, worthlessness, anxiety and fear. It can be very helpful to pay attention to these feelings as they can be harnessed to assist the clinician to express appropriate empathy.

ANXIETY DISORDERS

Anxiety is an emotion experienced as a normal phenomenon in response to threat or uncertainty. Anxiety disorders occur when anxiety is out of proportion to the threat posed and also impacts on the patient's functioning. The focus of the anxiety may be specific, for example particular phobias such as arachnophobia (fear of spiders), or may define the characteristics of the disorder, for example panic disorder (experiencing panic attacks and avoidance of situations that may precipitate these) and generalised anxiety disorder (experiencing a generalised sense of anxiety and worrying about being worried). Typically, anxiety disorders demonstrate links between thinking (cognitive symptoms such as being fearful of experiencing a heart attack in panic disorder), emotional response (symptoms of worry including physical symptoms) and behaviours such as avoidance of the feared object or situation or of safety behaviours (travelling with a paper bag in case of feelings of imminent sickness or of hyperventilation). For some patients, there will be a very specific precipitant or trigger to the anxiety symptoms – exploration of when the symptoms first started is necessary as part of the consultation.

During the consultation, making links between what the person is experiencing in terms of thinking, feeling and behaving in a real-life example can give the clinician a clearer diagnostic formulation and also build the therapeutic relationship with the patient and a sense of shared understanding of the patient's anxiety symptoms. Specific therapeutic techniques based on the connections between thoughts, feelings and behaviour and modifying these to reduce symptoms is the basis of cognitive behavioural therapy, one of the main treatment choices for anxiety disorders.

THE OVERLAP BETWEEN SYMPTOMS OF DEPRESSION AND ANXIETY

Anxiety and depression are recognised as discrete primary disorders. However, there is often some overlap between the two: most depressed patients also have some symptoms of anxiety, and many of those with more severe anxiety disorders will also have some feelings of depression. Enquiry about predominant experiences and concerns that the patient has is very important. Exploration should include presence of physical symptoms, such as sweating, increased heart rate or palpitations, frequency of micturition or opening of bowels, headache, and associated changes in functioning and activity, such as whether the patient has stopped usual enjoyable activities, including hobbies and socialising with friends. Changes in behaviour, for example increased smoking or use of alcohol, and cognitive symptoms, such as concerns of having a heart attack, fear of impending doom, worry about being worried and thoughts of hopelessness and a bleak future are also commonly present. Within the consultation, it is important for clinicians to elicit biological symptoms of depression, including the mood

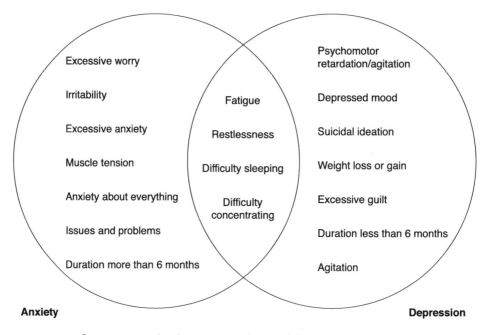

FIGURE 3.1 Symptom overlap between anxiety and depression

of the patient, particularly a diurnal variation with mornings being worse, and the impact on their daily lives of sleep, specifically early morning wakening, and changes in appetite, weight, libido and bowel function.

Visually, the overlapping symptoms of anxiety and depression can be summarised in a Venn diagram (*see* Figure 3.1).

Scenario

Jennifer Smith is 30 years old, single and works as a council project manager. She attends the GP surgery regarding persistent fatigue over the last 3 months – she is concerned that a 'virus', about a year ago, may be the cause of her problems. Despite feeling so tired, she is sleeping very poorly, including waking in the morning 2–3 hours earlier than usual. She is low in mood in the morning but feels a little brighter later on. She is tearful several times a day. Her appetite is impaired and she has lost around 5–6 kilograms in weight. She is seeing less of her friends – feeling too tired and not currently enjoying socialising. She has missed several days of work in the last month.

Generally she is fit and healthy – she is not on any prescribed medication. Her parents separated when she was 12 years old. She is an only child. Her mother, who works as a social worker, moved from Norwich to Edinburgh about a year ago. She lives with her partner of 14 years and his two teenage children. Until this move, her mother was close to Jennifer – seeing each other most days, being 'best friends' and going on holidays. Jennifer rarely sees her father, although he lives in Norwich – he is a distant and cold man. Her grandparents have all died – she sees little of the rest of her family.

Jennifer was born in London and moved to Norfolk when aged 10. Her parents often argued, only one of them wanting more children. When Jennifer was 13, her parents separated and her mother met her current partner 3 years later. Jennifer did well at school – a good athlete, had many friends and passed her A levels with good grades. She studied politics at London University. She found London lonely – she had few friends and used cannabis and other drugs regularly. Her studies suffered and she gained a lower-grade degree than expected.

She held a few clerical jobs and has worked as a Norwich Council project manager for the last 3 years. She initially was very happy in this job. However, in the last 6 months she has been less motivated and had less satisfaction from her work.

She had one boyfriend at university. This ended when he had an affair – for a few weeks afterwards she had vague suicidal thoughts. In the last couple of years, she has had a couple of brief relationships but is currently single.

She smokes 10 cigarettes a day. She drinks a bottle of wine, alone at home, one or two nights a week – although none in the last couple of months. She now rarely uses drugs – the last time was 6 months ago.

SKILLS FOR YOU TO APPLY
Establishing initial rapport

How you greet a patient who is overtly depressed is crucial. Matching the pace of their speech and mood and picking up and responding to verbal and non-verbal cues is a very important part of developing initial rapport. Look especially for facial expression and tone and pace of talk – try to match it.

Don't say:

Hello, tell me about your depression.

Try this instead:

Clinician: *Hello . . . Jennifer Smith? I'm X, a nurse with this team . . . What should I call you?*
Patient: *Um, Jennifer would be fine.*
Clinician: *Well Jennifer, your GP asked me to see you today . . . she is worried about your tiredness and that you have been off work for some days in the last month . . . I'd like to ask some questions to work out how I can help you . . . Can you tell me how you are feeling today?*

OR:

> Clinician: *Hello Miss Smith. I'm Dr Y, a doctor working in this team. Your GP has written to me as she is worried about your mood . . . Can you tell me a bit more about what's been happening to you recently?*

Listen, facilitate and gauge the patient's emotional state

Listen to the patient's opening statement without interruption, showing concern and compassion. Express empathy when appropriate and continue to pick up and respond to verbal and non-verbal cues.
Don't say:

> *Why do you say you're depressed?*

Try this instead:

> Clinician: *You have told me that you have had some days off work recently and that you are missing your mother . . . could you tell me a bit more about how this is making you feel at the moment?*

OR:

> Clinician: *What you have told me, about not sleeping at night, feeling tired all the time and being tearful, might make anyone feel down . . . could you tell me more about how you have been in the last couple of weeks?*

Open and closed questions

Direct the patient into an open question about feelings – this will often get you to the root of the problem more promptly. Allowing the patient to express feelings is often cathartic, although it is a question of careful timing when to signpost the interview into directive questions to enable the patient to tell more of the story and feel more in control. Directive questions about why the patient feels they are depressed, what the main concerns are, what the effects on personal life and work are and any hopes or expectations from the clinician are highly important.
Don't say:

> *Your GP says you've been anxious – is that right?* or *So you haven't been sleeping well recently?*

Try this instead:

Clinician: *You've said that you've felt anxious and low over the last few months . . . please tell me a bit more about that.*

OR:

Clinician: *You told me you aren't going to work some days . . . that you can't face it . . . that when you are there you can't concentrate . . . tell me more about this.*

OR:

Clinician: *Earlier you told me that you found London lonely. Is that right? . . .*
Patient: *Yes, very lonely.*
Clinician: *And you also mentioned that you were regularly taking street drugs. Is that so? . . .*
Patient: *Yes, that's right.*
Clinician: *Can you tell me a bit more about why you were feeling lonely and using drugs when living in London?*

Clarify

Repetition, paraphrasing and the use of silence all help to 'open up' a patient who is feeling hopeless, worthless and guilty.
Don't say:

Tell me about work?

Try this instead:

Clinician: *You've told me how difficult it is to sleep . . . I'd like to know more about this . . . what is going through your mind when you are awake in the night?*
Patient: *Oh, I just lie there and worry about why am I feeling like this? I keep on thinking about that virus I had a year or so ago. I'm sure that set it off. Then I just feel so awful I worry about how I am going to face tomorrow.*
Clinician: *Are you having difficulty getting off to sleep?*
Patient: *That's not too bad. It's usually later in the night I have problems.*
Clinician: *What happens later at night?*
Patient: *Well I wake up and I just can't get back to sleep.*
Clinician: *What time are you waking up?*
Patient: *Er, around 4, I guess. It varies a bit.*

Clinician: *4 a.m.? That is early. Is that a change from the time you usually wake up?*

Another example:

Clinician: *So, you had a boyfriend for about a year at university but this ended when he had a fling with someone else.*
Patient: *Yes. That was a bad time.*
Clinician: *A bad time?* (Clinician remains silent, allowing the patient to formulate her response.)
Patient: *Yes . . .* (Pause) *I actually felt so bad I started to think about killing myself. I just felt that I couldn't go on.*
Clinician: *Things must have been very bad for you to feel like that. Can you tell me a bit more about those thoughts of harming yourself at that time?*

Discover the patient's perspective

Directive questions about why the patient feels they are depressed, what the main concerns are, what the effect on personal life and work have been and any hopes or expectations from the clinician are important and may also help to clarify the story.

Don't say:

Tell me how your life has been affected by your problems?

Try this instead:

Clinician: *Are you able to rate this for me out of 10 (if 0 is the absolute lowest you could be and 10 the happiest)? Where would you rate yourself now?*
Patient: *Oh, pretty low. Say 3 out of 10.*
Clinician: *You've told me about how this has left you with poor concentration and little energy . . . how has it affected things at work?*
Patient: *I just can't get on there at present. I can't concentrate or take things in. It takes me ages to do even simple things and even then I make mistakes. I really struggle with meetings. Some days I just can't face going in at all.*
Clinician: *. . . and in your social life?*
Patient: *What social life? I don't have one any more. I'm so tired when I get home all I do is lie on the settee. My friends think I've given up on them.*
Clinician: *Jennifer, earlier you said you thought you'd had a virus which was causing your symptoms . . . can you tell me why you think it's a virus?*
Patient: *Well, I felt terrible about a year ago – aches and pains, headache, feeling all hot and cold – and the doctor said it was probably just a virus*

and it would get better itself. But when I started to feel really bad again I started to worry that the virus might have come back – or perhaps I've got something like ME. Someone at work has a friend who got ME and she ended up in bed for over a year!

Clinician: *. . . your doctor doesn't think it's a virus, and he hasn't found any other physical cause, so what else do you think could be causing your symptoms?*

Summarising

Using this skill at the end of a specific area of inquiry enables the clinician to confirm that they have understood what the patient has said and helps the patient feel the clinician is listening attentively to them. For example:

Clinician: *Let me recap what you have just told me . . . your parents separated when you were 12 . . . about a year ago your mother moved from Norwich to Edinburgh . . . you've always been very close to her with you regularly going out together with her being like your best friend . . . now she is further away, you have much less contact . . . your father still lives locally but you rarely see him . . . have I got this information right?*

OR:

Clinician: *So that I'm sure I've got what you've told me . . . you've been sleeping very poorly recently and felt very tired in the morning . . . some days you've felt too tired to go into work . . . other days, when you do go in, you've not been able to concentrate on tasks and have struggled in meetings . . . is this correct?*

Signposting

Structure can be provided by the clinician by using signposting to move the consultation to new areas of inquiry. For example:

Clinician: *We've talked a little about how you have been feeling recently . . . how it's affected your work and close friendships . . . I need to know about other areas of your life . . . such as your family, your time at school and at university . . . Could I now ask you to tell me about your parents?*

OR:

Clinician: *I want to ask you about your sleep, appetite and mood in a bit more detail in a minute but first, Jennifer, it would be useful if you could tell me more about your time at university in London . . . how did you find living in London?*

Demonstrate empathy

It is important to express empathy skilfully. Patients will quickly detect if your tone of voice does not match what you say. They may think, or even say, 'How can you know what I'm feeling?' Tears particularly require a supportive body language and empathy – and may also need touch, silence, the offer of a tissue and knowing when to move the consultation on.

When a patient is being tearful talking about their mother, don't say:

Let's move on to something else . . . would you tell me about your father?

Try this instead:

Clinician: *Whilst we've been together, I've noticed that you've been mainly looking at the floor and that when you do look at me, you look as though you are near to tears . . . Jennifer, it's important that you tell me how you've really been feeling recently . . .*

OR:

Clinician: *You told me that your parents separated when you were 12 years old and that your mother, to whom you have always been very close, moved to Edinburgh a year ago . . . I can appreciate that someone going through this might feel very low.*

Accept

Accepting non-judgementally what the patient says and how they feel is important, particularly if they do not feel deserving of care. Avoid premature reassurance.

Don't say:

You didn't do well at university . . . why was that? or *You'll soon be better . . . don't worry yourself.*

Try this instead:

Clinician: *I know you are feeling anxious and low now . . . but it is good you are seeking help.*

OR:

> Clinician: *I understand that it can feel embarrassing talking about your use of cannabis and other drugs . . . but it's important for me to know more about this.*

Provide support

Discover the patient's support systems and offer support yourself.
Don't say:

> *That's terrible. Now I want to talk about . . .*

Try this instead:

> Clinician: *It sounds as though you and your mother have been less close since she moved away . . . but I'm hearing that you have a couple of good friends who could be very supportive to you.*

OR:

> Clinician: *I understand you've been feeling low recently . . . I can see you feel very alone . . . but it is very good that you're seeking help and have come to see me today.*

Other examples of specific phrasing for uncovering depression and anxiety include:

➤ *You've told me that you feel hopeless and guilty about your situation . . . do you feel that you can be helped at all?*

➤ *You are wondering if you are depressed. I'd like to ask you some specific questions about your mood, appetite and sleeping patterns which will help me understand this a bit more . . .*

➤ *Do you ever feel that there's some light at the end of the tunnel . . . that you will get better?*

➤ *Some people feel that they can't go on when they are depressed . . . have you had thoughts like that? . . . that you'd like to end it all? . . . have you made any plans?*

➤ *Is there anything you've stopped doing since you've become unwell? . . . things that you don't feel you currently have the energy to do?*

➤ *Would you agree that you appear low at the moment?*

➤ *Would you be willing to accept some help? . . . whether that be by taking a suitable medication or talking through your difficulties with a trained therapist?*

TOP TIPS

After your opening question asking what has brought the patient to the consultation today, allow the patient to talk uninterrupted for the first minute.

Use the patient's own language when summarising and chunking and checking the information you have gathered thus far.

Use the patient's language when picking up on cues and signposting to allow further exploration of the Mental State Examination.

OSCE practice task 1

Philip Hall is a 27-year-old man who has presented to accident and emergency with symptoms of acute anxiety and concerns that he may be having a heart attack. Use appropriate Calgary–Cambridge skills to elicit symptoms of anxiety and come to a diagnostic formulation.

You have 10 minutes to perform the task.

OSCE practice task 2

Fred Rounce is a 73-year-old man who was widowed 6 months ago. His daughter, who is concerned about him, has brought him to the GP surgery. His main concern is his difficulty sleeping, although he has also lost 4 kg in weight.

Explore his concerns, including assessing whether he has symptoms of depression.

You have 10 minutes to perform the task.

FURTHER READING

Beck J. *Cognitive Behavior Therapy: basics and beyond.* New York, NY: Guilford Press; 1995.

Wells A. *Cognitive Therapy of Anxiety Disorders: a practical guide.* Chichester: Wiley; 1997.

CHAPTER 4

Assessing risk to self: suicide and self-harm

Ann Stanley

LEARNING OUTCOMES

- To be able to assess suicidal risk in a patient who has just harmed themselves using the Calgary–Cambridge model
- To communicate the findings of the assessment to the patient
- To identify the correct care pathway for the patient

INTRODUCTION

Suicide, attempted suicide and self-harm have become more frequent in recent years. Fifty years ago, suicide was illegal, leading to the risk of imprisonment if unsuccessful. The level rises and falls with available means. Legislation and industrial development have removed common means, for example: the move from town gas to natural gas in the 1970s, paracetamol and aspirin sales being limited in the 1990s and the introduction of catalytic converters to car exhaust systems in the 2000s. Suicide and self-harm are not of themselves mental illnesses; most people at some point in their life will think of suicide but only a few will act upon it. The purpose of assessment is to determine the nature of the intent, the presence of a mental illness and to arrive at an agreed care pathway with the patient. Good communication with this group of patients is required to achieve these outcomes.

The subject attracts many myths, perhaps the biggest one being that if you speak to a person about suicide, they will go away and kill themselves. In many cases the reverse is true and the individual is relieved to have the opportunity to talk about it. Conversely, it should be remembered that sometimes patients will underplay their intent to use the next opportunity to complete the act. It is the assessment of this intent and the patient's understanding of the risk that their chosen means presents which are key, rather than the actual risk. To give two alternative examples, I remember a lady in her 70s who had taken a small number of sleeping tablets (benzodiazepines) being sure they would kill her, and a 14-year-old admitted to the medical ward having taken a significant quantity of paracetamol (90 tablets or so) who was just wishing to make a cry for attention. I spoke with her mother, who said, 'It's only paracetamol', and was horrified when she realised that her daughter could have killed herself with the amount she had taken. The intent was far greater in the first case, although the risk was far greater in the second.

Whatever speciality of medicine you practice in, from time to time you will have to assess a patient who has harmed themselves. The deliberate self-harm rate is 400 per 100 000 population with a wide variation: 65–70 per 100 000 for men aged over 75 and 800–850 per 100 000 for women aged 15–24. An inner city accident and emergency department can expect to see around 200 patients following self-harm each month. The Calgary–Cambridge model provides the framework within which to carry out the assessment.

The framework will allow you to:
1   Frame the assessment in the light of the patient's own experience.
2   Build a relationship.
3   Determine their understanding of their actions.
4   Gather information about events to attempt to reach a shared understanding of the situation.
5   Agree on an action plan.

Demographic factors

The assessment of risk involves being aware of the demographic factors that are associated with an increased likelihood of completed suicide.

Risk factors for completed suicide relating to the individual

➤ Age – peaks in early adulthood (male) and following retirement (both genders)
➤ Gender – male > female
➤ Family history of suicide
➤ Poor physical health, chronic illnesses and pain
➤ Presence of mental illness, mental disorder – particularly depression – alcohol misuse and personality disorder
➤ Social isolation

➤ Unemployment, debts
➤ For those in employment, unskilled workers and professionals
➤ Singleton

Interviewing a patient after a self-harm/failed suicide attempt

The patient must be kept safe until they are fit to be interviewed. The length of time before this can happen will be dependent upon the method used. When the interview takes place, a quiet and private place needs to be chosen. Interruption should be kept to a minimum. Building a good rapport at the start of the interview is the key to making a good assessment. The patient may well not wish to speak with you. The greeting of the patient and the explanation of the purpose of the interview are very important for the further success of the assessment. It is necessary to check that they are comfortable and feel that their physical comforts have been considered. There must be no hint of a need to hurry.

SKILLS FOR YOU TO APPLY
Establishing a rapport

For both of these scenarios, the rapport with the patient is key. An opening statement introducing you to the patient and explaining the purpose of the assessment is essential. It is also important to establish what the patient wishes to get from the consultation.

➤ **Establish initial rapport** by greeting the patient and obtaining their name, e.g. *Hello, can I just confirm your name? What do you wish to be called?*
➤ **Introduce** yourself, role and nature of interview and obtain consent if necessary, e.g. *I am Dr X, I have been asked to see you by the team currently looking after you to assess how we can best help you following recent events. The information you give me will be kept confidential within the team.*
➤ **Demonstrate respect** and interest and attend to patient's physical comfort, e.g. *Are you comfortable?*
➤ **Identify the reason(s) for the consultation**
➤ **Identify** the patient's problems or the issues that the patient wishes to address with an appropriate **opening question**, e.g. *What problems brought you to the hospital?* or *What would you like to discuss today?*
➤ **Listen** attentively to the patient's opening statement, without interrupting or directing the patient's response, e.g.:
  – Scenario 1: *I understand that you have cut your wrist. Can you tell me about what happened?*
  – Scenario 2: *I understand you took some tablets. Can you tell me about the events leading up to you taking them?*
➤ **Confirm list and screen** for further problems, e.g. *You have told me about headaches and tiredness; anything else . . .? How are you feeling about it now?*

➤ **Negotiate agenda**, taking both patient's and physician's needs into account. Following self-harm/a suicide attempt, it is vital to screen for future risk of completing suicide and decide where the patient should be, e.g. at home, in hospital and what follow-up, if any, is required.

By the end of the interview, you will need to have established the method used, degree of planning and underlying mental state of the patient. The whole process is a risk assessment. In your head you are checking the risk factors, both demographic and relating to the individual attempt, using questions such as those earlier in the chapter.

The next step is to determine the issues that the patient wishes to address and the dialogue needs to start with an open question, e.g. *How do you see things now?* It is vital not to appear judgemental. You must allow the patient time to ventilate their feelings and discuss issues important to them – even if you feel that they are not relevant. Consider your use of vocabulary to minimise the possibility of misunderstandings; be aware of cultural and religious sensitivities. Once the rapport is developing, you can move on to the next stage – that of information gathering.

Clinician: *Can you tell me the events which led up to you being here?*

Remember a depressed person may be very slow in their responses. Try not to use multiple questions. Although the process will be slow, ask open rather than closed or leading questions.

Factors relating to the interview
➤ The patient's beliefs and feelings
 — *What did you expect from your overdose/self-harm?* The key thing is the patient's expectation of the risk to them rather than the real danger. *Was it painful? What was the pain like?* For some, it is a pleasurable experience which leads to a repeat of the behaviour. It is often worth exploring the patient's understanding of the effect on those close to them. *Have you thought how your mother, partner or children might feel about it if you were to end your life?*
➤ Surprise, anger, or bitterness at survival
 — *How do you feel now?* Subsequent questioning will be led by the tone of the answer. There may be surprise at the experience of the self-harm – *I didn't realise it would be that painful* – anger that they are still alive or a feeling of failure.
➤ Ongoing suicidal thinking, particularly where a clear plan is in mind
 — *How do you see the future now? Will you harm yourself again? What plans do you have?*

➤ Hopelessness is a key risk indicator
  — Patient: *I can't even do this successfully.*
  — Clinician: *What are you going to do now?*
➤ Non-verbal cues suggestive of suicidal intent
  — The patient may appear at peace with themselves. They may also have clear symptoms of depression with paucity of movement, slow speech at low volume and minimal eye contact.

Ongoing risk to self

People may self-harm for various reasons, including as a cry for help, a means of generating endorphins to give a feeling of well-being or a failed suicide attempt. After such an attempt, it is important to determine how the patient views the future. As part of the interview, the symptoms which put patients at risk need to be considered. Is the patient displaying depressive symptoms such as low mood, lack of motivation, sleep disturbance (in particular early morning wakening) and has their weight changed? Is there diurnal variation in mood? Hopelessness and worthlessness are very important symptoms for predicting future risk of completed suicide. *I am a failure, I can't even kill myself properly* is a not-uncommon manifestation. Self-harm can be both impulsive and planned. Minor impulsive episodes can go wrong, leading to unintended consequences. Anger and substance misuse – both alcohol and drugs – can all have a role. The symptoms have to be viewed in the light of the current presentation.

Questions need to be open and non-judgemental:

How *not* to do it:
Did you think taking an overdose was clever?
Do you realise that your cutting attempt has caused a mess?
I can see why you felt that no one likes you and that you are a failure. Why couldn't you have succeeded in your overdose?
Haven't you thought about the effect on anyone else?

A better way of doing it would be questions such as:

How do you feel about things now?
What areas are you concerned about?

The key is to spend the time to allow the patient to feel that they wish to speak with you, to open up to you, to move things forward. Having built up a rapport, the next step is to gather the necessary information to put together a view of the risk.

Information gathering

The patient's perception of the risk posed to him/her by the method of self-harm chosen is key, rather than the actual risk. The interview needs to determine the intent of the harm and the plans for the future.

Exploration of patient's problems

Encourages patient to tell the story of the problem(s) from when first started to the present in own words (clarifying reason for presenting now), e.g.:
- *When did you first have thoughts of harming yourself?*
- *What made you feel like that?*
- *How did you plan it?*

Uses open and closed questioning technique, appropriately moving from open to closed, e.g.:
- *Did you write a will? (closed question)*
- *What other plans did you make?*

Listens attentively, allowing patient to complete statements without interruption and leaving space for patient to think before answering or go on after pausing, e.g.:
- *How were you found?*
- *Were you expecting them to return?*

Facilitates patient's responses verbally and non-verbally – use of encouragement, silence, repetition, paraphrasing, interpretation, e.g.:
- *So what time did that happen?*

Picks up verbal and non–verbal **cues** (body language, speech, facial expression, affect); **checks out and acknowledges** as appropriate, e.g.:
- *I can see you are finding this difficult but it is really important for me to be clear as to what happened to help you. Can I just check that I have understood it correctly?*

Clarifies patient's statements that are unclear or need amplification, e.g.:
- *Could you explain what you mean by light headed?*
- *Can you explain why you needed to show that you loved her in this way?*

Periodically summarises to verify own understanding of what the patient has said; invites patient to correct interpretation or provide further information.

> **Uses** concise, **easily understood questions and comments**; avoids or adequately explains jargon. **Establishes dates and sequence** of events.
>   Actively **determines and appropriately explores**:
> - patient's **ideas** (i.e. beliefs re cause)
> - patient's **concerns** (i.e. worries regarding each problem)
> - patient's **expectations** (i.e. goals, what help the patient had expected for each problem)
> - effects: how each problem **affects** the patient's life
>
> **Encourages patient to express feelings**

ASSESSMENT OF SELF-HARM

The assessment of self-harm is an inexact science relating to both the assessment of the patient and an assessment of the risk. The latter is also hard to quantify, but there are clearly several factors that have been associated with suicide and with further self-harm. It is vital to be aware that self-harm is not itself a mental illness; in fact, thoughts of self-harm are probably so common at some point in life as to be considered a normal, albeit not universal, phenomenon. Nor is self-harm a reliable diagnostic sign of any given mental disorder, with great variation in the rates of mental illness reported from different studies of those who self-harm. It is, conversely, also relevant to consider that it is unlikely that anyone would self-harm who was not in some psychic distress (perhaps notwithstanding a couple of esoteric genetic disorders associated with idiosyncratic self-harming).

It is also important to note that the assessment of self-harm is fraught with the paradox of unreliable information. Self-harm that is intended to kill might be underplayed by the patient, whilst self-harm that is intended to express or discharge intolerable feelings might be presented in a very dramatic fashion. Often it is also the case that a seemingly insignificant self-harming event might have carried great suicidal intent, but little danger of actual loss of life. Only the patient will know what was intended by the act of self-harming.

A number of risk factors are presented hereafter that might be useful in distinguishing whether a high level of risk of subsequent suicide is present. The list is neither exhaustive nor universal, and does not equate to whether further self-harm will occur. In general, repetition is common, and any self-harm is a signal of an increased risk of subsequent suicide.

An awareness of other psychiatric diagnoses present that would increase risk is important.

There are a number of specific questions that you should consider asking:

➤ *Have you ever wished you weren't here/were dead?*
➤ *Have you ever thought about hurting or killing yourself?*

➤ *Have you ever acted on those feelings? (When, how, what precipitated each attempt? Was there an actual intent to die? Who rescued/found you? What treatment was obtained?)*

➤ *When is the last time you felt suicidal?*

➤ *Have you been feeling suicidal lately?*

➤ *How have you thought you might go about killing yourself?*

➤ *Do you currently have the means to carry out this plan (e.g. rope, pills or gun)?*

➤ *Do you have easy access to a gun? Is it at home? Is it loaded? (Always discuss guns with suicidal patients, even if they are not part of the divulged plan, because of their high lethality and frequent use in suicide.)*

➤ *How close have you come to actually carrying out this plan?*

➤ *Do you wish you were dead now?*

➤ *Have you thought about killing anyone else? (Homicidal and suicidal feelings often co-exist, and homicidal thoughts can be explored much like suicidal thoughts.)*

Factors relating to the act

In order to try to judge the risk for the future, it is important to be aware of factors directly related to the act. The factors listed below have been shown to be good indicators of future risk. It should be remembered that the risk is determined by the patient's perception of the risk rather than the actual risk.

➤ Planning
  — How far has the suicide planning gone?
  — Has a specific method been chosen?
     • Are the means available?
     • Has the sequence of events been thought through?
     • What is the wished for outcome – death, injury, attention from others?
  — Is the plan feasible? Is there a method?
  — How dangerous is the planned act?
  — Is the person likely to be found?

➤ Evidence of forethought in the act, complex and careful preparation
  — Has the person gathered the means?
  — Has there been a rehearsal?

➤ Final acts such as reparation of debts, making of wills, etc.

➤ Intent

➤ Clear belief that the act would/could kill

➤ Method

➤ Violent means traditionally thought to carry more risk

➤ An escalating pattern of attempts

➤ Setting

➤ Choice of isolated setting where discovery unlikely

What is the history of past behaviour?

It is important to know about previous attempts. A detailed description of the event itself, the events preceding it and what happened after would be vital in judging the current episode.

Factors relating to the interview

The purpose of the interview is to establish the patient's current feelings and view of the future. Now that they have survived, how are they going to move forward? The key point of the assessment is to have a view as to the risk in the near future. The factors listed below need to be explored in a sensitive way.

➤ The patient's beliefs and feelings
➤ Surprise, anger, or bitterness at survival
➤ Ongoing suicidal thinking, particularly where a clear plan is in mind
➤ Hopelessness

It is important to consider a number of questions after assessments of self-harm:

➤ What was/is the level of intent of the act?
➤ What were the reasons for the act/plan to self-harm?
➤ Is there a mental disorder underlying the act/presentation?
➤ What management is necessary?

The actively suicidal individual may not tell you the truth in that they may wish to go and complete the act. As a depressed patient gets better, they may discover the motivation to complete the act.

Once the assessment is complete and you have gathered the information which will lead you to the plan, you need to share the information with the patient. Key things to consider are where the patient is going to go and what support mechanisms are in place. The assessment of self-harm as compared with suicide is best demonstrated with contrasting scenarios.

Scenario 1: Assessment of self-harm

Darryl Hunt, aged 27, has presented to a local casualty department having cut his left wrist, repeatedly, with a broken bottle. He has been waiting in the department for several hours whilst his wounds were stitched and he has a hangover, and would rather be in bed. You have been asked to review his suicide risk and to decide if it is safe for him to leave hospital.

Yesterday evening Darryl had to drink after he and his girlfriend, Angela, had had a row. Later she had sent Darryl a text message threatening to leave him. Darryl went out in search of more to drink, but the barman refused to serve him as he was already intoxicated. He then called his girlfriend and told her that he was in town and that if she didn't forgive him, then he would cut his wrists.

Angela put the phone down and so he grabbed a bottle from a wall, smashed it, and cut his wrist vigorously three or four times. He was shocked by the amount of bleeding, and called his mum, who took him to A&E.

Darryl has no previous history of mental health problems or self-harm. He currently lives with his mother and has a job in a supermarket. He has been going out with Angela for several months and thinks she is 'the best thing that ever happened to me'. He believes they will settle down together and doesn't know how he could cope if she ever left him.

He feels rather ashamed of his behaviour, but is relieved (and also quite proud) that Angela has come to the hospital and has been waiting with him. He thinks the hospital are 'making a fuss' and just wants to go home.

Suggested questions:
How do you see things now?
Do you have any further plans to harm yourself?
Will you be safe at home with Angela and your mother?
How else could you have responded to the situation?
Can you think of another way to tell Angela how important she is?

Scenario 2: Assessment of suicide

Mr Bert Ramsay (age 73) was admitted to the medical admissions unit yesterday following an overdose of nitrazepam. Two days ago he took a full box of tablets. The medication had belonged to Maud (his wife), who died 6 months ago. Following her death, Mr Ramsay had put the tablets aside 'just in case I might need to end it all'. Subsequently he had ruminated on taking the pills for the next few months, usually waking early in darkness to mentally plan his death. He hasn't been eating well, and has lost interest in most of his usual activities. For the last 2 weeks he has thought of little else, and has gone to bed hoping he would die in his sleep, as he felt unable to face the next day. He had spent a week or so planning this suicide in detail; had cancelled the milk and put the cat into a cattery. He waited until his daughter had made her monthly visit before posting a couple of second-class letters to her and his son in Australia. He pulled the curtains, put on his favourite dark suit, tidied the house and took the pills one by one until there were none left. His memory of the next few hours is pretty hazy, and he can't recall how he came into hospital. According to the ward nursing staff, the postman had attempted to deliver a parcel the following day, and was shocked to find the curtains closed and that Mr Ramsay did not answer the bell. It seems he called the police, who broke down the door and then rushed him into hospital by ambulance.

Mr Ramsay thought he would die from the overdose. He thinks his life has little value. He feels a total failure; ashamed that he failed to kill himself and angry that he is still alive. He feels completely hopeless and that he is a total waste of everyone's time. He still wants to die and has thoughts about doing so by attaching a hosepipe to his car exhaust.

Suggested questions:
What did you think would be the outcome of the overdose?
How do you feel about the future?
Do you have any further plans?
Would you be safe being at home?
Do you think you might be depressed?
Have you thought about coming into hospital?

Arriving at a shared understanding

At the end of the interview, you as the clinician need to be clear whether you are happy for the patient to go home. Using the two scenarios above, Darryl will go home with his mother and partner. Bert has only an empty house to return to, his attempt was well planned and he is bereaved and depressed. He has a very high likelihood of repeating the attempt unless he is treated and support put in place. Had I assessed him, I would be admitting him, I would hope informally, but if he refused I would consider using the Mental Health Act 1983 (as amended in 2007).

OSCE practice task 3

In 10 minutes, using one of the scenarios above:
1 Establish the method used for self-harm.
2 Explore the planning of the episode of self-harm.
3 Investigate the likelihood of a repeat.

FURTHER READING

Gelder M, Andreason N, Lopez-Ibor J, *et al. New Oxford Textbook of Psychiatry.* 2nd ed. Oxford: Oxford University Press; 2009.

Stein G, Wilkinson G. *Seminars in General Adult Psychiatry.* 2nd ed. London: Royal College of Psychiatrists; 2007.

University of Manchester. *National Confidential Inquiry into Suicide and Homicide* [Annual Report]. University of Manchester; July 2010.

CHAPTER 5

Information gathering in psychosis

Jaap Hamelijnk, Andrew Tarbuck and Somayya Kajee

LEARNING OUTCOMES

- To understand how to establish a rapport with a psychotic patient, develop a shared understanding and negotiate an agenda regarding the purpose of the meeting and its outcome
- To know how to assess abnormalities of thought, perception and insight in patients with psychosis by using both the Calgary–Cambridge model and the Mental State Exam
- To be able to explore psychotic patients' symptoms, beliefs and understanding of their experiences in order to establish a working diagnosis

INTRODUCTION

Managing patients with psychosis is a core task for professionals working in mental health services. Often these patients are the hardest to communicate with as they may be out of touch with reality or suffer with delusions and/or hallucinations that can make them mistrustful and uncooperative. This in turn may result in poor communication and consequent difficulty in building a rapport. Patients presenting with a psychotic illness can vary greatly in their symptoms, from being very acutely unwell with thought disorder to being very guarded with much more subtle signs.

Although patients with psychosis will usually end up under the care of mental health services, a significant number of them will initially present in other clinical settings, such as primary care or accident and emergency. Recognising that a patient has a psychotic illness can be difficult, particularly in the early or prodromal stages of the illness. These difficulties are made worse if the patient is paranoid, suspicious or reluctant to engage in the assessment process. The stigma associated with mental health problems can also affect both patients and staff, and professionals need to overcome this. Good communication skills are, therefore, vital in order to work effectively with such patients and conquer these difficulties.

Research with patients suffering from a first psychotic episode has highlighted the importance of early detection and shown how this can have a significant impact on treatment outcome (Marshall *et al*, 2005). The psychoses (e.g. bipolar disorder and schizophrenia) are among the 20 leading causes of disability in the world, with the highest incidence amongst young people (Murray and Lopez, 1996). It is, therefore, extremely important that all clinicians can recognise psychotic symptoms and understand how to work with such patients. The importance of early intervention and treatment in psychosis is now well recognised because they are clearly linked to improved outcomes. The initial presentations are key times in assessing and accessing help, and research shows people with psychosis present to various agencies on average eight times before they receive help and that help is often up to 18 months after their initial symptoms start.

The first few minutes of the consultation are crucial, as this will usually determine the tone for the rest of the meeting. An attempt has to be made to establish trust and build rapport with someone who may not be there willingly or may not believe they are unwell. The challenge for the clinician is to negotiate through all these difficulties while still doing the crucial job of gathering information about their psychosis, making sense of the patient's and their family's difficulties and then relaying this back to them before discussing management. Thus there will understandably be anxiety from both the patient and clinician. The clinician will have to use a wide range of communication skills and techniques, like open questioning and recognising non-verbal cues, and undertake this in an empathetic and non-judgemental way. If this first meeting is negotiated successfully, it can set the scene for further meetings with both the family and patient where they feel understood and listened to.

This chapter looks at applying the Calgary–Cambridge guide in patients presenting with psychotic symptoms; highlighting those skills that may be of particular help in establishing this very important first contact, or for maintaining a therapeutic relationship with established patients. Students can be very fearful of talking with psychotic patients and often do not know how to approach either the patient or the problem. The key is to apply the Calgary–Cambridge guide and, if necessary, modify the skills. One of the most important skills is patience; a calm, unhurried and interested attitude towards the patient is vital, listening to the patient's story as it unfolds. Patients with a psychotic illness generally function poorly and are aware of having severe difficulties. Giving the patient time and space to explore how help can be offered is very important. To establish a diagnosis, more detailed information is often required. This chapter will also discuss some of the skills that allow the clinician to make a detailed exploration of symptoms whilst maintaining a meaningful therapeutic relationship.

SKILLS FOR YOU TO APPLY
Preparation

Chapter 2 describes the information and preparation needed before the interview takes place. Patients with psychosis can be unpredictable, or even occasionally potentially dangerous, and it is impossible to conduct an interview well unless you feel safe and secure. When patients present with a psychotic disorder, they may need to be able to sit further away from others; psychosis can affect the size of personal space. Discuss the referral with other team members beforehand and decide who needs to be present for the consultation and who will take the lead.

Sometimes the consultation takes place at the patient's home. In these situations it is even more important to negotiate its purpose. Gaining entry to a patient's own home can be difficult. The fact that you made the effort to go and see the patient is important in building the relationship. However, when the patient has previous experience of psychiatric services, they may be aware of the significance of the home visit and know that you may be considering interventions the patient may not want (for example, the use of the Mental Health Act). Under these latter circumstances, the assessment may have been requested by a third party (such as a social worker, approved mental health professional or the patient's family) and the patient may have been totally unaware of the visit prior to your arrival. Whilst there is still a clear need for an explanation of who you are and what you are doing there, if the patient is thought-disordered or paranoid, a full explanation of your mental health role may immediately increase suspicion and impair rapport.

Introductions

Introducing yourself and explaining why you are there is essential. Make sure the patient has understood who you are and that you know how to address the patient. At this point, it is necessary to clarify the reasons for the consultation and negotiate the purpose of the interview carefully. Patients do not always seek help themselves and are sometimes brought to the clinic by others. It is very helpful to be aware of this situation as it may have an impact on the building of the relationship and prevent the clinician from being seen as colluding with the carer or others. However, the fact that the patient has attended is a positive feature and suggests that he is likely to want help of some sort.

Gathering information

Listening to the patient's story is very important. Do not 'leap in' too early with direct questions. Pay attention to any non-verbal cues displayed by the patient, as these can help you to assess their emotional state. However, it is not always appropriate to overtly respond to them; reflecting back verbal or non-verbal cues immediately can induce irritability, tension and suspicion. It is often helpful in building a rapport to ask first about 'external' problems (i.e. how their life is being affected) rather than initially focusing on 'internal' problems (i.e. the symptoms themselves and the patient's emotional reaction to them). The aim is to develop a shared understanding of the patient's perspective and beliefs – acknowledging them and showing empathy but without colluding in the patient's illness.

Flexibility with regard to questioning is essential. In particular, it may be necessary to move between open and closed questions or reverse the open-closed cone. Clarification is also vital. Psychotic patients often make statements that are vague, unqualified or ambiguous, and you should make sure that you have clearly understood what the patient is saying. It is particularly important to clarify if the patient really is describing particular psychopathological symptoms (e.g. thought insertion), as these can have particular diagnostic significance.

It is often very helpful to obtain accurate information from a third party or informant (such as a relative, friend or another professional) who knows the patient well and can describe recent changes in their behaviour and emotional state. This can be perceived as threatening and unsupportive to a paranoid person with disordered thinking; if the doctor is aiming to achieve a collaborative relationship, it is good to have the patient's permission if possible. In these circumstances, relatives and friends are often anxious and sometimes angry, which may also complicate the interviewing process. It may be necessary to allow extra time to talk with the patient's family, who may naturally be overwhelmed by what is happening to their relative. Under some circumstances, it may be appropriate to ask for others' views without the patient's knowledge. It is always acceptable to listen to what carers wish to tell you. Always be sensitive with third-party information; disclosure to the patient could put the informant in a difficult position, or even occasionally at risk.

Building the relationship

Ensure that you display appropriate non-verbal behaviour throughout the interview. Remain calm and avoid too much movement. Be flexible with regard to eye contact; some paranoid patients find direct eye contact threatening and it may increase agitation. Try not to show surprise and remain non-judgemental. Be very careful with the use of touch and humour; both can easily be misinterpreted and are probably best avoided in psychotic patients.

Try to show empathy if possible, but beware of being insincere as this can easily destroy the rapport that you have worked hard to develop throughout the consultation. The aim is to show non-judgemental acceptance and understanding of the patient's position and hence offer appropriate help but without colluding in their illness.

Structuring the interview

Careful signposting and summarising can be very helpful techniques with psychotic patients. These patients are often very disorganised in the way they present information, for example as a result of poor concentration or thought disorder. Providing a structure for the patient and checking the accuracy of their views can be calming and reassuring.

Scenario

The patient is a student at university. He believes that he is being psychologically tested and made to look mad because he has found solutions to previously unsolved mathematical conundrums. He thinks that the lecturers at the university are trying to steal them to claim his work as their own. This started with lecturers giving him lower marks for coursework. The patient has noticed them talking about him in code and looking at him in a strange way. There are coded messages on TV and in newspapers. The patient can hear them talking about him via telepathy. They comment on what he does. The patient felt he was being monitored through his TV and so he threw it away, but despite this he still has the experience of feeling spied upon. The patient feels he is being followed, but his friends deny that this is the case. The patient has confronted people in the street about this and his friends have told him not to be so stupid.

All of the patient's time is spent in his room researching these issues; his thesis is behind as he can't concentrate on it. He cannot sleep, has no time to eat and has lost weight. He feels anxious most of the time and at times believes that he is in real physical danger.

HOW TO DO IT

The key tasks are:

➤ identifying the reasons for the consultation and negotiating an agenda
➤ gathering information
➤ talking about delusions and hallucinations
➤ handling difficult questions and requests
➤ the assessment of insight.

Identifying the reasons for the consultation and negotiating an agenda

It is very important to establish the reasons for the consultation early in the interview process. It is likely that the clinician's agenda is very different from that of the patient. Negotiating a common ground for the consultation and how the patient could gain benefit from it is an essential skill. Listening to and carefully clarifying all the areas in which the patient would like help will provide the basis for the consultation and the cooperation of the patient. When others are present, it is important to clarify the agenda of all those in attendance. It helps to be patient with introducing the clinician's agenda; first emphasise how you can be helpful to the patient and then present your agenda from the patient's point of view, avoiding the use of jargon.

Don't say:

I've been asked to see you because your friends think you are mentally ill!

OR:

*Your tutor thinks you may be paranoid and deluded, so I have come to see
if we need to treat you with antipsychotic medication!*

Try this instead:

Clinician: *I hear that you are not eating or sleeping very well and seem to be
'stressed out'. Perhaps we could see if there is something that can be done
to improve things? I also wonder if it would be helpful to talk a bit about
how worried people are about you and how things may have been difficult
for you recently? In order to do this, I would like to hear your story in more
detail and perhaps get to know you a bit better? Then we can discuss how
we can work together and make you feel a bit better. Does that sound OK
to you?*

Patient: *There's nothing wrong with me! I've just got so tired that I can't
concentrate because of everything that is going on.*

Clinician: *It certainly sounds like you are having a difficult time and are very
stressed. Perhaps we could start off by talking about that?*

Using words like 'we' and 'us' will create the impression you want to work with the patient and draw the patient into a dialogue. The aim is to develop a dialogue in which it is safe to explore difficult experiences or thoughts.

Gathering information

Eliciting psychotic symptoms can be very challenging for the interviewer. The patient may be very reluctant to reveal any information that could put him in a difficult situation or lead to admission to hospital. Open questions that you would normally use early in an interview (such as: *Could you tell me how you have been feeling recently?*) may produce little response. You may need to try a variety of approaches if the patient does not follow your lead and 'open up'; for example, try an educated guess to clarify the situation. Once you have the patient's trust, and they are willing to talk, you can follow the patient's lead and ask further clarifying questions which link and make sense to him or her.

Signposting is essential in guiding the patient and reducing any fear the patient may have about the interview, for example:

> *I would like to talk a bit more about worries you have . . .*
> *To help me understand better what has been troubling you, can you say a*
>   *bit more about . . .*

You can help build rapport by first exploring the patient's 'external' problems (the patient's concerns regarding the effect on their life) rather than 'internal' symptoms. If the patient becomes agitated, carefully moving from more threatening 'internal' problems to less threatening 'external' problems can be helpful. You will be able to return and clarify 'internal' symptoms in due course, weaving in and out as required.

Don't say:

> Clinician: *Tell me how you have been feeling recently.*
> Patient: *Er, well, that's difficult to say, really . . .*
> Clinician: *Well, what has been worrying you?*
> Patient: *Lots of things . . .*
> Clinician: *Such as?*
> Patient: *Things going on here at the university.*
> Clinician: *What do you think might be going on?*
> Patient: *I don't think it might be going on; I know that this is happening!*
> Clinician: *But what exactly are you talking about?*

Try this instead:

> Clinician: *I understand that you are studying at the university. Perhaps I*
>   *could start by asking you about how your course is going?*
> Patient: *Well, it was going OK to start with, but then . . . well, things started*
>   *happening, you know . . .*
> Clinician: *And has that affected your work?*
> Patient: *Well, I think my work is fine, but the tutors started to give me lousy*
>   *marks. I didn't understand at first, but then it became clear that this was*
>   *all part of the 'test'.*
> Clinician: *The 'test'?*

Patient: *Yes. You see, they found out that I had worked out how to solve the problem, which they didn't like, because they thought that they should have solved it first. And now, they don't want me here and have got it in for me . . .*

Clinician: *When you say 'they', do you mean your tutors?*

Patient: *Yes; well, them and others in the department.* (patient getting angry and agitated)

Clinician: *This sounds very stressful. Has it affected you in other ways? Are you able to sleep all right, for example?* (changing to less threatening topic)

Patient: *No, I can't sleep or eat properly. I can never relax, even in bed, because they won't let me!*

Patients with psychosis may find it difficult to talk about emotions or recognise emotions accurately. In schizophrenia, emotional responses may be blunted or incongruous, which means out of keeping with the expected response given the topic under discussion, whilst seemingly neutral topics may lead to paradoxically intense responses. If the patient does get agitated or distressed, acknowledge that you have touched upon a difficult area and ask if the patient would prefer to leave that particular topic, at least for now. Carefully summarising the story back to the patient and signposting what the clinician needs to discover next may calm the patient, particularly when used in conjunction with offers of help.

Other symptoms (like formal thought disorder) are observed, rather than asked for. Giving the patient the opportunity to talk and listening to their speech is very important. The interviewer needs to adopt the 'interested listener' approach by being calm, sitting still, taking time and being attentive to the patient.

The patient may not think they are 'ill' (i.e. they may lack insight). Under these circumstances, the clinician needs to reflect back the patient's experiences and develop a shared understanding from the patient's perspective of how these experiences are affecting their life.

Talking about delusions and hallucinations

By definition, psychotic symptoms such as delusions and hallucinations are not viewed by those experiencing them as being 'unreal'. As a rule, the patient is very preoccupied by their content, but may initially be reluctant to discuss their experiences for fear of being labelled as 'mad' or because of fear (e.g. concern that the clinician may be 'part of the conspiracy' – *see* 'How to handle difficult situations' on page 53). Often, once you are able to break through this initial reluctance, patients are very keen to discuss the beliefs and experiences that have become the major preoccupation of their life.

Record any beliefs expressed by the patient accurately and clarify the exact nature of the phenomena they are describing. For example, if the patient talks about hearing voices, it is very important to gather as much information as possible about them (e.g. how many voices are there, is it one voice or several, where do they appear to come from, do they comment on what the patient is doing, are they talking *to* the patient in the second person or are they talking *about* the patient in the third person?). It is tremendously helpful if the patient can provide examples of what they are experiencing. These should be written down verbatim in the health record. Time also needs to be given to exploring and recording the *evidence on which abnormal beliefs are based*. It may be the only time that the patient discloses this information, which may have very significant diagnostic implications.

Attempts to assess the extent of the patient's thoughts, beliefs and thinking processes can be difficult and requires judicial use of open and closed questions. Try reversing the 'open-to-closed cone' by asking a closed question first, followed by more open questions to clarify the symptom carefully. Linking the symptom to a specific situation is helpful in getting the exact detail.

Example:

Clinician: *Have there been situations when you heard the voices of people around you although there was nobody there?* (closed question)

Patient: *Yes, at nights, in my room. They are talking, all the time, trying to distract me and keep me awake so that I'll fail in the 'task'.*

Clinician: *Where do the voices come from?*

Patient: *I'm not exactly sure. At first I thought it was from the corridor or the room next door, but I've searched them and they aren't there. I think it may be something to do with telepathy. I know one of them has friends in the psychology department, so he knows all about mind games . . .*

Clinician: *How many voices are there?*

Patient: *Lots! They are all involved!*

Clinician: *Do you recognise their voices?*

Patient: *Mostly members of the faculty.*

Clinician: *What do they say?*

Patient: *Horrible things. They aren't true; they are trying to drive me away so they can say I've failed and steal my work.*

Clinician: *Can you give me an example of exactly what they have said?*

Patient: *Well, last night Professor Smith kept on saying, 'He's become too great a risk, we have to get rid of him!' and my tutor said, 'It won't be long now before we break him!'*

Beware of taking things at their apparent face value without clarifying and exploring symptoms as fully as possible. For example, consider the following.

Don't say:

Clinician: *Have you ever had the experience of people putting thoughts in your head?*

Patient: *Well, yes, I think that happens quite often really.*

(Clinician writes 'patient has thought insertion' in the case notes.)

Try this instead:

Clinician: *Have you ever had the experience of people putting thoughts in your head?*

Patient: *Well, yes, I think that happens quite often really.*

Clinician: *Could you tell me a bit more about that and perhaps give me an example?*

Patient: *OK. I was watching a programme on TV last night and during the commercial break there was an advertisement for a new video game. I thought it looked really good and so I decided to buy it this morning.*

Clinician: *You're talking about the power of advertising?*

Patient: *Yes. That's right.*

Having clarified the patient's initial statement, it becomes clear that the patient is not describing the Schneiderian first-rank symptom of 'thought insertion'!

How to handle difficult situations

'Why are you writing notes?'

Whilst many patients have concerns about the confidentiality of medical information, this may be a particular issue in dealing with psychotic patients. Paranoid patients may be very upset if you start taking notes in the interview. Sometimes they can be reassured by your explanation regarding why you are writing things down and how they will be part of the confidential medical record. However, some patients will not accept this and there may be no alternative but to record nothing at the time of the interview itself and write the case notes up afterwards.

Patients sometimes ask to see what has been written about them. Patients do have a right of access to their medical records and they can apply formally to the NHS Trust. However, you may share your own notes with the patient if you feel it appropriate to do so, and indeed many clinicians now ask patients if they would like to receive a copy of the letter written to their GP. However, you should not allow patients to see notes written by other clinicians without obtaining their permission and you must be particularly careful with regard to third-party information.

Although medical information is confidential, there are circumstances in which information has to be shared, either within the multidisciplinary team as part of clinical management, or sometimes with outside entities such as approved mental health practitioners, social services and sometimes the police or the courts. Where possible, the patient should be informed of any obvious need for information sharing from the outset (e.g. if the patient is being seen for a court report) and caution is required if a patient requests a 'blanket agreement' with regard to confidentiality.

'Are you in with them?'

Paranoid patients are desperately trying to make sense of the changed and frightening world in which they find themselves. Sometimes they believe they are caught up in some form of conspiracy and do not know who to trust. They often wish to share information with others who will believe them and assist them in taking 'appropriate action' (e.g. involving the police, security services, etc.). But how do they know if they can trust you?

Such concerns can give rise to a variety of 'difficult' questions or statements, such as:

➤ *I think you are part of the plot!*
➤ *How do I know if I can trust you?*
➤ *If I tell you, how do I know you won't pass it on to them?*
➤ *You do believe me, don't you?*

It can be very difficult, and sometimes impossible, to satisfy the patient about such issues. Being clear that you are a health professional working as part of the NHS and reminding the patient of your earlier stated position regarding confidentiality (see above) may help. Beware of 'locking horns' with the patient, belittling their ideas, colluding or making promises that you cannot keep.

What not to say:

Patient: *How do I know that you won't tell them everything I am saying to you? Are you in with Professor Smith and that lot?*
Clinician: *Don't be silly. Of course I'm not 'in with them'!*
Patient: *Could you go to the police about this then? They wouldn't believe me, but if you could convince them it's true . . .*
Clinician: *Of course I will. But first, you need to tell me as much as you can about it.*

Try this instead:

Patient: *How do I know that you won't tell them everything I am saying to you? Are you in with Professor Smith and that lot?*
Clinician: *I'm a clinician. I don't work for the university and I don't have anything to do with the university. I can see how difficult things are for*

*you at present and what I want to do is help you feel less stressed and help
you to cope better.*

Patient: *Do you believe what I have told you?*

Clinician: *I can certainly understand why you are feeling so upset and
distressed.*

Patient: *Could you go to the police about this then? They wouldn't believe
me, but if you could convince them it's true . . .*

Clinician: *Before we decide how best to help, it would really be very useful
if we could be as clear as possible about what you have experienced. Is
that OK?*

It is important not to confront delusions as false beliefs – empathise with the
patient's situation and legitimise their experience without necessarily agreeing or colluding with their interpretation of reality. Offering explanations that
accept the patient's experiences as valid and showing empathy but providing an
alternative view is a difficult balancing act with a psychotic patient, particularly
if they challenge you and ask you if you think that they are mad. It is helpful
for the clinician to find phrases that work well in different circumstances and
to practice them. Do not rebuff, but remain interested in their view and offer
empathy and help with their problems. Remember that although the patient
may be very ambivalent about whether or not to talk with you, there is often a
strong underlying drive to share these very important thoughts with someone.
Given patience, sufficient time and an appropriate approach, many patients will
gradually 'open up'.

The assessment of insight

Insight is often a very poorly understood concept. It is not an 'all or nothing'
phenomenon that is either 'present' or 'absent'. It is really a complex set of beliefs
that relate to the patient's understanding of their situation, symptoms, illness,
treatment and their relationship with society. The assessment of insight is valuable, however, as it does provide information about whether or not a patient is
likely to accept the need for treatment or remain concordant with medication.
A measure of the importance of insight can easily be obtained by inspecting
the statements written on section papers of patients detained under the Mental
Health Act. You will very frequently find statements such as, ' . . . the patient lacks
insight and refuses to accept the need for hospital admission'. Lack of insight is
thus often being invoked as a core reason for depriving mentally unwell patients
of their liberty – a powerful concept indeed!

Listening to the patient's perspective of their problems, picking up their non-
verbal cues and asking sensitively how they are feeling may give you information
not only about the content of the patient's symptoms but also about the extent

of their delusions or hallucinations, their emotional reaction to them and how firmly they believe in them. Openly challenging or contradicting a patient's view of psychotic symptoms will be counterproductive and destroy the rapport that you have worked so hard to build up. However, it may sometimes be appropriate to gently explore the degree of conviction that a patient has.

Example:

Patient: *When I'm in the university library, I know they are watching me. They have some form of rota; sometimes one faculty member is there, sometimes another. They stare at me.*

Clinician: *Might it just be coincidence? For example, could they just be there working?*

Patient: *No! I thought about that. But I started to keep a chart, noting down who was there each day. There is a clear pattern to it. They are definitely spying on me.*

OSCE practice task 4

You have been asked to see Mr Robert Smith (age 29), an unemployed administrative assistant who lives alone in a council flat. He has become increasingly socially isolated in recent months. There have been several increasingly acrimonious exchanges with his neighbours, in which Mr Smith has accused them of 'bugging' his flat and 'tapping' his telephone. The police have become involved because of complaints from both Mr Smith and his neighbours regarding one another's behaviour.

Your task is to take a history from Mr Smith regarding the recent problems he has experienced and to clarify the exact psychopathological features he describes.

You do not need to discuss treatment options with the patient.

In the last minute, you will discuss the case with the assessor.

You have 10 minutes for this station.

REFERENCES

Marshall M, Lewis S, Lockwood A, *et al.* Association between duration of untreated psychosis and outcome in cohorts of first-episode patients: a systematic review. *Arch Gen Psychiat.* 2005; **62**: 975–83.

Murray C, Lopez A. *The Global Burden of Disease.* Harvard, CT: Harvard University Press; 1996.

CHAPTER 6

Information giving and shared decision making in psychosis

Katherine Hill, Jonathan Wilson and Ann Stanley

LEARNING OUTCOMES

- To be able to discuss an initial management plan with a psychotic patient involving referral to secondary care, psychological and pharmacological treatment options
- Explain to a patient the reasons for medication, its side effects and mode of action
- To explain the rationale for a Mental Health Act assessment to a patient where this is necessary

INTRODUCTION

Although the management of psychosis is generally within the remit of mental health services, all clinicians will encounter people with early psychosis. GPs will occasionally see new cases, A&E staff will often see people with an early psychosis presenting with self-harm, help-seeking or bizarre behaviour related to their psychotic beliefs, and surgeons will see patients with dysmorphophobic symptoms.

Assessment skills have been discussed in Chapter 5. In this chapter, we take the assessment on a stage further into developing an early management plan at whatever level that is possible and referral on to appropriate help. Different skills are needed for ongoing work with people with psychotic symptoms, and these are outside the remit of this book.

These same skills will also be transferable to other spheres of medicine where there may be disagreement between patients and clinicians about the diagnosis, nature of the problems, therapeutic goals or negotiating an agreed treatment plan. As such, it is a useful communication skill to practice.

SKILLS FOR YOU TO APPLY

In this section you will need to:
➤ explore the effects of the patient's experiences on their life
➤ their understanding of the nature of these experiences
➤ gather information in a way that leads to areas of possible agreement and manage disagreement
➤ be able to talk about mental illness and psychotic illness and symptoms in a way that is not frightening and alienating to patients
➤ be able to discuss initial therapeutic options where there is some agreement
➤ discuss your concerns and management where agreement cannot be reached
➤ maintain rapport throughout!

To achieve this, we have highlighted key skills from the guide which will need applying with greater depth, intention and intensity.

The scenario is to be found in Chapter 5 (page 48).

HOW TO DO IT

What is different in negotiating and agreeing a treatment plan with a psychotic patient in general terms?

The key tasks are:
1 Develop a shared rationale for an early management plan.
2 Explain the rationale for the initial management plan.
3 Be able to discuss antipsychotic medication with a willing patient.
4 Be able to explain the need for a Mental Health Act assessment to a patient in whom this is required.

Task 1: Develop a shared rationale for an early management plan
Developing rapport
It is important to accept the legitimacy of the patient's views and feelings and to remain non-judgemental. For example:

Clinician: *I can see that it is all very distressing for you.*
Patient: *They are just mean, giving me low marks. It is because they do not want me to find the solution and they know that I am nearly there.*
Clinician: *Low marks always seem hard. Can you tell me what it is that you are near to solving?*

AND:

> Clinician: *I think you said earlier that you were feeling tired and so were finding other things difficult. Would looking at your sleep be a good place to start?*
>
> Patient: *I can't sleep because I have lots of things to do and I have to make notes of my solution.*

Additional skills for understanding the patient's perspective

It is necessary to actively determine and explore the following:

➤ patient's ideas (i.e. beliefs re cause)
➤ patient's concerns (i.e. worries) regarding each problem
➤ patient's expectations (i.e. goals, what help the patient had expected for each problem)
➤ effects – how each problem affects the patient's life.

And encourage the patient to express their feelings:

> Clinician: *It must be very difficult for you if you think people are talking about you all the time?*

Achieving a shared understanding; incorporating the patient's perspective

In order to do this, it is important to:

➤ Relate explanations to the patient's illness framework and to previously elicited ideas, concerns and expectations.
➤ Provide opportunities and encourage the patient to contribute by asking questions, seeking clarification or expressing doubts. The clinician then needs to respond appropriately.
➤ Pick up verbal and non-verbal cues (e.g. that patients need to contribute information or ask questions, are experiencing information overload or distress).
➤ Elicit patient's beliefs, reactions and feelings regarding information given and terms used. Where appropriate, these need to be acknowledged and addressed.

Unlike in other areas of medicine, in psychosis one cannot assume that patient and clinician have a similar understanding of the nature of the problem and, therefore, the treatments or help required. This has to be actively worked at. To be able to move on to discussing a management plan rather than just eliciting symptoms, the interviewer has to prepare the ground first by exploring the patient's views of their problems (ideas, concerns and expectations) and their openness to alternative hypotheses or viewpoints. Rather than offering certainties, the clinician offers possibilities or opinions and actively seeks the patient's views verbally and through non-verbal cues to gauge the effect. In doing this, you hope to identify areas of agreement of problems that can be the focus of a developing treatment plan and manage areas of disagreement. From this, you aim to develop a shared language to discuss their difficulties that reflect the patient's views of their problems yet also reflect your views.

In this example, exploring the belief doesn't lead to much consensus or feeling of shared understanding.

Discussion of coping strategies to this point can be useful in seeing what strategies the patient uses and to what level they have been successful. These can then be built upon in engaging the patient in a management plan. If the patient has been coping with voices by distracting themselves with music or activity, this can be explained and supported as a legitimate coping strategy. However, if the voices at times cannot be managed in this way, then that could be a route into discussing alternative strategies that services can offer, including the use of medication to try and settle the voices.

Although psychotic patients can be perceived as being uncooperative and lacking insight, in practice there may be many areas of agreement and concern that may be shared. Early on in the psychotic illness, patients are often much more open to the possibility of other causes for their experiences and are actively questioning and testing out possibilities. A patient will often accept that they are distressed rather than ill. Working with the patient on these areas can lead to the development of an initial management plan and engagement with services. Here it is worth tentatively exploring their beliefs about these experiences and their openness to alternative views.

> Clinician: *Colin, you said that you can hear your lecturers in your room and yet you cannot see them. How is that possible, do you think?*
> Patient: *I think it's via telepathy. They might also have bugs.*
> Clinician: *Do you generally believe in telepathy?*
> Patient: *I didn't before, thought that Paul McKenna stuff was all phony. But now I do.*
> Clinician: *Generally I understand telepathy to be reading people's minds rather than hearing someone's voice.*
> Patient: *Yeah, that's what I thought, but . . .*
> Clinician: *Is it possible you could be mishearing noises, such as from the TV or radio, and because you're worried about your course you're reading your worries into it?*
> Patient: *I don't know, it seems so clear but my friends can't hear it.*

In this example, the patient is perplexed and is thinking about different possibilities. In other circumstances, they may completely disagree. Where there is some openness, there is room to offer alternative views of their difficulties, such as suggesting your own interpretation to see what they feel about this.

> Clinician: *Sometimes I see people who are under a lot of stress. When the stress gets very high and they're not sleeping or eating, that can sometimes lead to their brains playing tricks on them. We know that people in solitary confinement, for example, start to see and hear things that are not there. I wonder if it's possible that with all the stress you are under and the lack of sleep this could be happening to you?*

Remember, however, that the purpose of this questioning at this stage is only to come to some shared agreement that there may be a mental health issue that requires help or treatment, not to challenge their underlying belief system in the way that cognitive behaviour therapy for psychosis may do!

It is often later in the course of their illness, as the delusional beliefs 'crystallise out' and become fixed, that patients may become less amenable to discussion as their delusions become immutable. It is possible to use good communication skills and explore all the above and still not come to a shared understanding. At this point, rather than endlessly arguing or persuading, the interviewer should graciously agree to differ on opinions. We will address how to do this and, at the same time, still manage the patient in the last section of this chapter. However, it is still worthwhile remembering that their experience of the interview and of the interviewer will affect the level of trust in services. A very bad experience can colour that person's perception forever. So even if a shared understanding cannot be obtained, a good interview that develops rapport and understands the patient's perspective is still worthwhile in terms of engagement and future work. Even if they do not accept it at this point, it sows a seed of possibilities of other explanations, or of a different viewpoint, that can be built on later. In seeming to have failed, one can have succeeded.

Out of these explorations and discussions in most instances (the exception being someone who is very unwell), the patient and doctor can usually find some common ground. This is what is called a *shared understanding of the nature of the problems*. It is the distress or difficulties arising from their experiences or beliefs that the patient would like to change or accept help with. In the second part of this chapter, we will move on to discussing what might be helpful for the patient. If rapport has been reasonable, both sides will have areas where they may disagree about the nature or significance of events, but in this context both can respect the other's viewpoint and work on the shared ground.

Task 2: Explain the rationale for the initial management plan
Planning shared decision making

To help achieve this, the clinician shares their own thinking as appropriate (e.g. their ideas, thought processes and dilemmas regarding the patient's condition and treatment).

The clinician involves the patient by making suggestions rather than directives and the patient is encouraged to contribute their thoughts – ideas, suggestions and preferences.

The goal is jointly to negotiate a mutually acceptable plan which offers choices and encourages the patient to make choices and decisions to the level that they wish.

The process concludes with the clinician checking with the patient if they accept the plan and confirming that their concerns have been addressed. The severity of the patient's illness may mean that the clinician has a professional view as to the minimum amount of help that the patient should have.

Items for consideration:
➤ Is medication needed?
➤ Would talking therapies be beneficial?
➤ Are substance misuse or physical health problems an issue?
➤ Is home treatment or inpatient care required?
➤ When does the patient need to be seen again?

Negotiating a mutual plan of action

In this part of the consultation, it will be necessary to:
1 Discuss the appropriate management options available (e.g. no action, investigations, medication, non-drug treatments).
2 Provide information on action or treatment offered; that is:
   — name of the medication
   — steps involved, how it works
   — benefits and advantages
   — possible side effects.
3 Obtain the patient's view of the need for action, perceived benefits, barriers to accepting and their motivation.
4 Accept the patient's views but put forward an alternative viewpoint as necessary.
5 Elicit the patient's reactions and concerns about plans and treatments, including their acceptability.
6 Take the patient's lifestyle, beliefs, cultural background and abilities into consideration.
7 Encourage the patient to be involved in implementing the plans, to take responsibility and be self-reliant.

8 Ask about the patient's support systems and discuss other available support.
9 Consider whether there is a carer involved and what information they need. Listen to any information they give or concerns they raise.

You should now have some thoughts regarding:
➤ the patient's problems
➤ your own 'bottom line' with regard to treatment
➤ some areas of agreement about the patient's problems
➤ some areas of disagreement.

It is worth summarising these and explaining how they are to be dealt with.

In preparation for this task, you will need to have clear in your head some terminology and a model for psychotic illnesses that you can use to explain to the patient. Schizophrenia is a term that carries enormous stigma and stereotypes, with press-fuelled images of mad axe-wielding people. In the minds of many people, this would be considered worse than having cancer. Hence this scenario also requires communications skills techniques regarding breaking bad news (*see* Chapter 10).

The early intervention model for all people with a first psychotic illness offers a structure for information giving that may be helpful to this scenario. Firstly, rather than diagnose schizophrenia straight off, the model suggests a diagnosis of *psychotic symptoms*. These can arise in the context of many different situations and illnesses: extreme stress, organic conditions, drug intoxication or withdrawal, affective disorders and also the psychotic illnesses (of which schizophrenia is one). It also uses a stress vulnerability model in which some people are more vulnerable or may become vulnerable in certain situations. When first assessed, information needs to be gathered and investigations performed to clarify which situation is the most likely. In the early stages of mental illness, there is a degree of development and a change of likely diagnosis is not uncommon, for example people can present with depression first, then develop schizophrenic symptoms later. A bipolar patient may present with depression but then develop a manic episode afterwards. Some diagnostic uncertainty at first meeting is inevitable and rather than commit to one diagnosis at this stage it can be helpful to be open with the patient about this and see part of the initial management as developing a better understanding of their problems and the likely causes. As such, this can allow discussion of symptoms and allusion to possible causes without having to feel a pressure to talk about schizophrenia. Some may see this as a 'cop out'.

Clinician: *Colin, you seem very stressed because you believe your lecturers are against you. You have said you can't sleep and aren't eating properly.*

You are also worried about your thesis because it's hard to concentrate. I am concerned about your mental health at the moment and how you are coping. I appreciate that you feel certain about everything you have told me. However, as you know, I wonder if you are reading too much into things you are hearing?

Then you need to discuss the options for management. For most people with a psychotic illness, referral on to a psychiatric team is the usual practice. If you have developed good rapport, and the risks are not too high, a general practitioner might chose to see the patient again or initiate some treatment which could be symptomatic (e.g. night sedation to help with sleeping) or could be more definitive (e.g. an antipsychotic medication). We will discuss the latter in the next section.

The level of discussions will depend enormously on what has been achieved in the first task and the patient's ability to accept alternative viewpoints or not.

Don't say:

Clinician: *I think that all your problems are due to the fact that you are mad and this is confirmed by you not agreeing with me. You need to see the mental health team.*

Try this instead:

Clinician: *I would like you to see a psychiatrist who could help you make sense of what's happening, which is clearly distressing. As you have said, you are having some experiences (such as hearing people when they don't seem to be there) that you can't explain and which may be a sign of mental health problems. Are you happy that I get in touch with them and ask them to see you?*

OR:

Clinician: *Colin, we disagree on what might be going on currently, but we do agree that you are under significant stress and finding it hard to cope. I think it would be helpful to refer you to a more expert colleague, a psychiatrist who can discuss what is happening further. Would you be willing to see them at least once to discuss with them so they can advise me?*

Remember, in the scenarios envisaged we are not expecting you to be a specialist in mental health, but rather a clinician who would initiate appropriate treatment and then refer on to appropriate services.

Task 3: Be able to discuss antipsychotic medication with a willing patient

In sharing the information with the patient, it is important to give the information in stages and check that the patient has understood it and applied it to their own symptoms. The patient will then be able to ask about their concerns.

You will need to be familiar with:

➤ one antipsychotic appropriate for initiating treatment
➤ describing to the patient how it works
➤ explaining what positive effects you expect it to have and over what timescale
➤ explaining common and important side effects and how these can be managed.

The positive effect you may expect to see and that which the patient expects to happen may be different. For example, you may want hallucinations and delusions to disappear, but the patient wants to feel less stressed and sleep better. They may not see there is a problem with hallucinations, as to them they are real experiences. This leads to the problem of clinicians feeling that medication is working, but patients feeling that it isn't because they are looking at different desired outcomes. Negotiating this successfully comes back to being clear about what are shared objectives and what are areas of disagreement for treatment and addressing both of those in explanations about effects and desired timescales. You should individualise the information to suit the patient.

It is important to be clear about the timescale of expected improvement, again with reference to possible different desired outcomes. Whilst antipsychotic effects take some weeks to develop, sedation and calming occur more rapidly.

It is helpful to try and include the most likely side effects and also those that are rarer but important (e.g. a reaction that means they should seek immediate help or stop the medication). A sense of the common side effects comes with practice rather than through reading the BNF. Novices can ask supervisors what in their clinical practice are the common side effects.

The example on risperidone below has been written in a fairly user-friendly style, but ideally you would want to personalise it further in order to relate it to the patient in front of you. You may also want to experiment with finding phrases and explanations that you feel comfortable with.

Example of talking about the side effects of risperidone medication:

Clinician: *There is a naturally occurring chemical in the brain called dopamine, which is involved with thinking, emotions, behaviour and perception. In some illnesses, this may be overactive and upset the normal balance of the chemicals in the brain. This excess chemical helps to produce some of the symptoms of the illness. The main effect that risperidone has is to correct the imbalance. This reduces the symptoms.*

Colin: *What do you mean 'symptoms'?*

Clinician: *You have described difficulty in sleeping and a change in your appetite. You believe that your lecturers are picking on you and talking about you. You are clearly stressed and distressed. The risperidone can reduce these feelings.*

Colin: *All medications have side effects, so what will the risperidone do?*

Clinician: *Some of the effects of risperidone appear soon after taking it, for example drowsiness. The most important action, however, to help reduce the symptoms of your illness, may take a few weeks of regular medication to become fully effective. People sometimes experience headaches or feelings of restlessness. It can also lower your blood pressure, so you might feel light-headed when you stand up suddenly. Some people may put on weight or experience problems with their sex life. Rarely, people get palpitations or skin rashes. Do not be worried by this list of side effects. You may get none at all. If you feel you have these or any other side effects, tell your doctor about it the next time you meet them.*

Task 4: Be able to explain the need for a Mental Health Act assessment to a patient in whom this is required

Discussing opinion and significance

This is a task in gently disagreeing, standing your ground about the reasons for this and being willing to explain them, and the necessity of this approach whilst trying to maintain some sort of empathy and relationship with the patient. Patients have described this as being to psychiatry what the decision to ventilate a patient is to acute medicine. When this is handled badly, the patient remembers it is as a very traumatic event, yet if handled sensitively there is scope for a working relationship after the event and many patients are grateful for the action taking.

The risk here is of being drawn into never-ending discussions, with clinician and patient trying to convince the other that they are right. It is fine to discuss your different viewpoints in order to influence the patient's decision, but there does come a point where it becomes clear that neither of you are going to change your opinion. This is not necessarily a point of ill feeling; it should be possible to agree that you both disagree.

The Mental Health Act 1983 (as amended in 2007) allows for patients with severe mental health problems to be admitted to hospital when they are unable to give consent or refuse to go. The admission of the patient should be the least restrictive way of managing the situation. Detention under the Mental Health Act provides safeguards to the patient. The grounds for detention are:

➤ the patient suffers from a mental disorder of a nature and degree to warrant admission to hospital
➤ that the patient needs assessment/treatment in hospital in the interests of one or more of the following:
  — their own health
  — risk to themselves
  — risk to others.

The next step is to determine their ability and willingness to consider an alternative view, namely your own or that of the 'medical model' of psychiatric illness. Essentially you will be:
➤ explicitly expressing the opinion that they have mental health problems
➤ explaining why you believe that, by naming and explaining their delusional beliefs and hallucinations
➤ explaining why treatment is needed, and then
➤ eliciting their response and reactions to this.

In this scenario, attempts at suggesting alternative views and approaches to the patient will at some point leave the interviewer clear that there is very little or no substantial ground for agreement of a shared management plan that adequately addresses the concerns of the clinician. The task then switches to informing the patient of the need to proceed to a Mental Health Act assessment.

The minimum level of information to convey is probably:
➤ an explicit acknowledgement of their concerns and views of the problem
➤ an expression of a different view of the problem that you hold and the reasons for this
➤ an explanation of the level of concern you have about the problem
➤ an explanation of your duty to ask for a Mental Health Act assessment
➤ an explanation of the process by which that will occur.

Clinician: *I know that you believe that the course tutors are against you and that legal action against them seems the only course open to you. I am concerned, however, that you may be experiencing mental health problems.*
Patient: *Are you saying it's all in my head?*
Clinician: *No, there may well be problems with the tutors, but I suspect that under the stress and lack of sleep you are under, your mind may be playing tricks on you.*
Patient: *What do you mean by 'tricks'?*
Clinician: *When you can hear your tutors but they are not in the room with you, I think that could be your mind playing tricks on you – what we call hallucinations – hearing someone's voice even when they are not there*

and there is no other rational explanation. I am very concerned because you are not eating as you feel you are being poisoned and are at risk of becoming physically weak and unwell. I believe you need help. Since you are not willing to have treatment, it is my duty of care to you to ask for a Mental Health Act assessment. Another doctor and approved mental health practitioner will meet with you to see if they agree with me that you are unwell and need treatment.

This may well be a repetition in part of your previous discussion as to your view. Here, however, it should be stated firmly and you should take control of the interview for long enough to state your opinion. It offers a last opportunity to enter into negotiation.

Arranging a Mental Health Act assessment

1 Phone the social services local access number and give basic information – usually, name, address, date of birth and nearest relative.
2 An approved Mental Health Practitioner (AMHP) contacts you and discusses the need for a Mental Health Act assessment. If necessary, arranges a second doctor.
3 All parties meet at an arranged place – patient's home, doctors' surgery, etc., and interview the patient.
4 Fill in paperwork.
5 Approved Mental Health Practitioner arranges transport to hospital and takes paperwork to hospital.

OSCE practice task 5

1 Having been given key symptoms of a patient's illness, explore their under-standing of the nature or explanation for these, their willingness to accept it as a mental health problem and take medication.
2 Explain to a willing patient the mode of action for antipsychotics and their side effects.
3 Given the key symptoms for a patient with psychosis, explain to a par-tially insightful patient why a referral to a psychiatrist is necessary in your opinion.
4 Explain to a distressed relative why a mental health act assessment is necessary on their son and how this will happen. You will be given the key symptoms and risk issues.

CHAPTER 7

Working with families and young people

Xavier Coll and Sarah Maxwell

LEARNING OUTCOMES

- To be able to use the appropriate skills for taking a family history; identifying who the patient considers as his/her family, clarifying the history of the different relationships, strengths and weaknesses of the relationships, coping mechanisms, communication patterns and the unmet needs of the individuals in the relationships
- To achieve a shared understanding of the information revealed during the session, integrating diverging opinions and negotiating between the parties, in order to be able to formulate a plan of action and close the session
- To equip clinicians with the skills needed to deal effectively with conflict, difficult behaviours and other complex situations encountered in working with families, such as deadlocks and secrets

INTRODUCTION

Why is this an important chapter for a clinician?

The underlying principles of working with families and groups of people are of great use in our daily clinical practice. However, even experienced clinicians can feel caught in the middle of complex relationship dynamics. The skills described in this chapter will help you to work successfully with family groups, especially if there are unspoken subjects ('secrets') between family members and/or beliefs that may influence those of your patient.

Working with young people is one of the few instances in clinical practice when doctors do not deal directly with adults. Adult medicine often consists of adult clinicians communicating with other adults, who share largely similar social values and norms about health, even when taking into account cultural differences.

Ill health can destabilise relationships or create a closer bond. Factors such as the nature of the mental health problem, the recognition (or not) that the problem exists, previous personal and family experience of coping with difficulties, the expectations of different family members and the vulnerabilities or resilience of each member of the group will determine the reactions. This is relevant because in addition to the potentially difficult dynamics, the clinician will also need to be aware of the rapid physical, psychological and social changes that take place in adolescence.

During adolescence, young people will develop new cognitive skills (including abstract thinking capacities), develop a clearer sense of personal and sexual identity, and move towards emotional, personal and financial independence from their parents. The professional's challenge is to maintain an effective clinical relationship while the health responsibilities transfer from the parents to the young person. The clinician must do this without undermining the confidence and competence of the relatives, engaging the group (not just the young person or the parents) and managing issues of adherence with the management plan, consent, confidentiality and the potentially strained relationships between young people and their families.

In this chapter, we will explore ways to facilitate our clinical interactions with children, young people and groups using the framework of the Calgary–Cambridge (CC) model (Kurtz *et al.*, 2005).

SKILLS FOR YOU TO APPLY

The CC model does not address the issues involved in the assessment of difficult family and group dynamics directly. However, it does address the issue of communicating with children and parents.

There are five phases in CC skills for this area, working with children over a spread of age and level of maturity:
1 Preparing and establishing initial rapport
2 Gathering information
3 Summarising and signposting
4 Explaining and planning
5 Closing the session.

1 **Preparing and establishing initial rapport**. Here, it is crucial to:
  — Create an appropriate environment for the child and the family, including toys and books appropriate to the age of the child or young

person, although some clinicians consider that they can be distracting, unless one is intending to use them.

— Pay attention to seating arrangements and greetings, establishing identities of the adults and children present.

— Engage the child through play (for a young child), neutral chat or by establishing rapport with the parents.

— Gauge the child's initial comfort level with you and adjust your approach accordingly.

— Start the interview by addressing the child and do not direct all your attention to the parent(s)/carer(s).

— Remember that the child is the patient but the parent is also a key person.

— Establish from the child or young person, if possible, who will lead on the story and how others will contribute (i.e. will the child or the parent start?).

— Establish interest, concern and attend to comfort of all members of the group.

2 Then, we should move on to **gathering information**, trying to:

— Ask young children whether they would like to tell their story or prefer their parents to do so.

— Acknowledge parental concerns and expectations during a consultation.

— Stop parents interrupting their children during interviews, whilst still acknowledging any disagreements.

— Actively encourage a shopping list of problems in the child's and parents' own words, using open and closed questioning techniques that are appropriate to the age of the child (closed questioning with choices tends to work well with young children; narrative with older children and young people).

— Determine and acknowledge the different ideas present in the group, since beliefs about the cause of illness may differ between parents and child or young person, and establishing both the parents' and child's perspectives, where appropriate, will assist us later on.

— Encourage the expression of feelings. Parents may be able to describe a young child's feelings, but it is valuable to provide space for young people to describe their own.

— If appropriate, take pregnancy, birth, immunisation, childhood illness, development, drug and allergy, family and social histories. This can work very well alongside drawing a family tree or genogram.

— When working with families and groups, it pays to gather information in the following areas:
  • history of the relationship
  • goals of the individuals in the relationship

- coping mechanisms that have been successful and unsuccessful
- precipitants for seeking treatment and/or assessment (*why now?* or *what has changed?* questions)
- communication patterns, both constructive and destructive
- description of the strengths and weaknesses of the relationship
- unmet needs of the individuals in the relationship.

3   Then, we need to structure the interview by **summarising and signposting**, especially when transferring attention from the child or young person to the parents and back again.
   — An example would be: *Kevin, your mother has just told me about your worries and what she thinks they are. Now I want to hear from you; can you tell me what is bothering you?*
   — Negotiate separate time with both teenager and parent/s. It is important not to marginalise teenagers. Valuing children and respecting their views is more likely to encourage the development of successful relationships between clinician and young person.
   — Consider asking younger children what they would do with three wishes or with a magic wand.

4   With regard to **explaining and planning**, we ought to:
   — Provide the correct amount and type of information suitable for any member of the family to understand.
   — Consider enrolling the parents to explain to a younger child on your behalf.
   — Incorporate the parents' and children's perspectives when giving information.
   — If appropriate, involve parents, children and young people in decision making.
   — Be aware of the different developmental needs of different age groups, with toddlers being naturally fearful of new environments and strangers, pre-adolescents being very private and self-conscious and teenagers even more so.
   — Offer children and young people opportunities to be involved fully in the information gathering and planning stages of the consultation.
   — Have a focus on initiating the interview, building the relationship and establishing rapport, which will ensure the patient's comfort and assurance throughout the consultation, paving the way for what may be difficult conversations later on.
   — If there is a need for a physical examination, it is important to create an appropriate environment for examination, being opportunistic and using the least invasive examination technique first.

5   Finally, when **closing the session**, it is important to make sure that the patient and the rest of the group feel heard and understand the mechanisms that the

clinician has put in place to ensure safety and maximise the benefits of the treatment plan – what is commonly referred to as a safety net. This appears to be the key to conquering parental and patient satisfaction, to ensure an accurate understanding and to reduce the power gap between a child or young person and his/her doctor, so that we facilitate effective communication.

Scenario

Kevin Smith, 16, is the eldest of five siblings. He has an 11-year-old sister, Suzie, and three brothers: Nathan (8), Connor (2) and Darryl (6 months). They all live with their mother (Chloe Smith), who is 32 years old and unmarried. Kevin was referred to his local Child and Adolescent Mental Health Service (CAMHS) by his GP as Chloe was finding his behaviour impossible to manage and was feeling 'at the end of her tether'.

Chloe and Kevin are seen as outpatients in their local CAMHS. Kevin has a long history of frequent outbursts. He has a reputation for being a loner, starting fights and hurting his peers. At school, he is disruptive, easily distracted and academically behind.

Kevin has symptoms of low mood and tends to ruminate on various ideas. This is worsened by the fact that he has very little contact with his peers, but leads an intense 'virtual' life through the Internet and inside his head. Kevin has been accessing pornographic websites involving minors when alone in his bedroom.

Kevin has self-harmed in the past, making superficial cuts to his forearms. He takes an active part in Internet chat rooms with people who say they have in common an interest in harming themselves.

Chloe recalls her own childhood as quite chaotic. She did not like school and drifted out of the school system at the age of 14, when she met Wayne, 4 years older than her. Wayne used to drink too much and was violent towards her. Their relationship lasted, on and off, 5 years. Wayne had been in trouble with the police, as he tended to 'get involved in fights'. Wayne is the father of Kevin and Suzie, but Kevin has not seen him for about 10 years. Nathan, Connor and Darryl all have different fathers. Chloe has a boyfriend, Carl, but he does not live with them. Chloe receives benefits, but money is 'tight'.

At home, Kevin feels close to Connor, who idealises him. Kevin, at times, takes care of Connor when Chloe is busy with Darryl. Kevin likes his mother, but resents that she has never given him much time. When Kevin was younger, he had to spend some time with his maternal grandparents, because his mother had drug problems (children's services were involved because of child protection issues).

In the scenario presented to you, the following aspects and dynamics within the family are likely to be very relevant:

➤ a complicated and convoluted family history
➤ Chloe and Kevin not really agreeing on what 'the problem' is
➤ Kevin having resentments towards his mother
➤ Kevin presenting with certain behaviours and thoughts that his mother is not aware of.

HOW TO DO IT

The key tasks are:

1 to identify who our patient considers his/her family, taking a family history of this scenario, describing the problem and its history, and establishing the importance of each member of the group
2 to achieve a shared understanding of the issues working with Kevin, integrating diverging opinions, negotiating between Kevin and Chloe, agreeing that there are difficulties and that we need a further appointment to both continue with the assessment and clarify the many strands of this case
3 to draw your own family tree and then Kevin's family tree
4 to identify communication difficulties that can affect adherence with the treatment when dealing with groups of people, such as dealing with a deadlock
5 to identify communication difficulties in relationships, such as the one between Chloe and Kevin; for instance, how to deal with secrets and the fact that Kevin is entrapped in his own thinking patterns and has become unable to engage with his peers.

Task 1: Identify who 'the family' is and establish the 'weight' of each member

It is important to avoid making assumptions about which people our patient will identify as family and about his/her home environment, since a patient can name a relative who is not a blood relation, a partner of the same sex or a close friend. Questions such as:

➤ *Who else knows that you are here today?*
➤ *Who do you call family? / Who do you regard as your family?*
➤ *Who lives with you at home? How long have they lived there?*
➤ *Do you have your own room?*
➤ *To whom are you closest at home?* Might help instead of *Do you get along with your mum and dad?*

Once family members have been identified, or while gathering information about the family, you could draw a family tree (Task 3 below).

Having gathered details about the family, you can add the patient's views on the quality of these relationships and whether there are problems that may affect the patient and their management. The following questions might help to explore these issues:

➤ *Kevin, who cares for you and takes responsibility for you?*
➤ *If you were upset or frightened, who would look after you and make sure that you were all right?*
➤ *If you do something well, who would be proud and praise you?*
➤ *How long have you lived where you live now, and how many times have you moved home in the last year or so?*
➤ *What is it like to live in the area that you do?*
➤ *What is the best thing about living where you do?* and *What is the worst thing about living where you do?*
➤ *Is there anyone else who ought to know you are here today?*
➤ *Have you tried to keep in touch with your father? What happened?*
➤ *Who is the most worried about you? How do you know?*
➤ *How do you think your mother sees you managing?*
➤ *Imagine someone treated you unfairly – what would you do?*
➤ *Think of a really good time you enjoyed with your family. What was it, and what made it so special for you?*
➤ *Other than your family, who is important to you in your life?*
➤ *At home, who is working and what do they do?*
➤ *Does your mother work away from home or at night, such that when you see her she is very tired?*
➤ *Is there enough money, from work and benefits, to meet your family's needs?*

In essence, the family can have a very significant influence on the care and the treatment that someone receives, no matter their age, because a person who experiences mental health problems does not do so in a social vacuum. Instead, their concerns about the course and outcome of their problems are usually influenced by their previous experience, by the illnesses of their family and friends, and by commonly held beliefs about the specific illness. These will in turn be influenced by the nature of the condition, which will determine the level of care, the length of time for which care will be needed and how predictable these care needs will be.

Relationships in every family, no matter how rigid or stuck they may appear, are dynamic and complex. At times of ill health, each person's capacity to adapt is tested, and relationships very often become more tense and uncertain. This is why it is often important to address other family members' beliefs and experiences of mental illness. These could be explored by formulating some of the following questions:

➤ *Has anyone in the family suffered from a similar problem?*

➤ *Who finds it most difficult to cope?*

➤ *Kevin, what does your mum think is the matter with you?* Or *Chloe, what brought you to see your GP about Kevin?* In essence, we ask different members of the family what ideas they have about the problems that the patient suffers from.

➤ *Kevin, when someone is ill at home, whose views about health and treatments are most influential in your family?*

Task 2: Working with young people

All the 'skills for you to apply' described earlier in this chapter will come to good use when attempting to formulate the issues of cases such as the one described here, and trying to reach a shared understanding of the main issues. When working with young people, we need to be aware of the challenges that they have to face. Particularly important are the development of a personal identity and intimate relationships with an appropriate peer, the establishment of independence and autonomy, the process of challenging authority, taking risks (such as experimenting with drugs, alcohol and relationships), seeking spiritual paths, changing schools and educational environment, and the transition from education to getting a job.

Here is a list of questions that might help when interviewing young people and their families that have not been covered yet in this chapter or in other chapters of this book:

When considering school and educational aspects:

➤ *Kevin, what school or college do you go to? How regularly do you attend?*

➤ *What are your favourite/least favourite subjects in school?* (instead of *How are you doing in school?*)

➤ *What might stop you going to school/college?*

➤ *What do you want to do long term?* Or *What do you hope that learning will help you do?*

➤ *Tell me about your friends at school*

➤ *Have you ever been suspended/expelled from school?*

To explore the activities interesting the young person:

➤ *Kevin, what do you enjoy doing with your family?*

➤ *What do you do for fun?* and asking to elaborate on the answers (instead of *Do you do anything outside of school?*)

➤ *What kind of hobbies (or activities) do you like doing best?*

➤ *When your mum is unwell, do you have to help to look after her or one of your brothers or sister?*

➤ *Are your friends mostly the same age as you, or are they mostly younger or older than you?*

➤ *How do you know that the people that you meet in the Internet chat rooms are who they say they are? Does it bother you? Do you meet them in real life sometimes?*

When enquiring about drug use:
➤ *Does anyone in your family smoke?*
➤ *Do any of your friends use drugs or alcohol?* (takes the focus away from the young person)
➤ *What kind of drugs have you seen around in your school or at parties?* (instead of *Do you do drugs?*)
➤ *Are you aware if drugs are bought and sold in your neighbourhood?*
➤ *Do you ever drink alcohol or use drugs when you are alone?*
➤ *Do you ever use alcohol or drugs to relax?*
➤ *Do you forget things you did while using drugs or alcohol?*
➤ *Do your family and friends ever tell you that you should cut down on your drinking or drug use?*

To find out about sexuality:
➤ *You said you have been going out with _____ for the last 3 months. Has your relationship become sexual?* (would follow naturally from information already provided to you in an otherwise difficult subject to approach)
➤ *Are you interested in boys/girls?*
➤ *Are your sexual experiences enjoyable?* (instead of *Have you ever had sex?*)
➤ *Have you ever been pressured or forced into doing something of a sexual nature that you did not want to do?*
➤ *Have you ever been touched sexually in a way that you did not want?*

On interview, Kevin describes ruminating over the idea of going into school and harming others. When seen on his own, Kevin makes reference to a 'plan' that would free the world of what he considers to be 'bad people' and create a better world. On further questioning, it appears that Kevin's idea of 'bad people' involves foreigners and immigrants.

Kevin also admits to thinking about bringing a fake gun into school and pointing it at the face of someone in the playground. He describes a sense of power and a certain amount of excitement over the idea that he could create an hysterical scene amongst other people, and have a powerful and significant role to play in this.

When asking about suicide, self-harm, and issues of safety:
➤ *When you are frustrated, angry or upset, how would people around you know that something was wrong?*

➤ *Have you ever thought about hurting yourself or someone else?*
➤ *Have you ever had to hurt yourself (cutting yourself, for example) to calm down or feel better?* (instead of *Do you cut yourself?*)
➤ *Have you ever tried to kill yourself?*
➤ *Violent behaviour seems to have become more frequent for many young people. Have you ever felt unsafe at home, at school, in your neighbourhood, in a relationship, or on a date?* (use one question at a time depending on the scenario)
➤ *Is any violence going on at home or at school?*
➤ *Have you got into physical fights in school or in your neighbourhood?*
➤ *Have you ever felt that you had to carry a knife or any other weapon to protect yourself?*

Finally, these could be five top tips when working with young people:
➤ See young people by themselves as well as with their parents. Do not exclude parents completely, but make it clear that the adolescent is the centre of the consultation.
➤ Be empathic, respectful and non-judgemental, particularly when discussing behaviours such as substance misuse that may result in harm, assuring confidentiality but knowing when to break it.
➤ Be yourself. Do not try to be cool. Young people want you to be their clinician, not their friend.
➤ Try to communicate and explain concepts in a manner appropriate to their development. For children and young adolescents, use only 'here and now', concrete examples and avoid abstract concepts ('if . . . then . . .' discussions).
➤ If appropriate, take a full adolescent psychosocial history (the HEEAADSSS protocol is helpful for this – *see* Appendix 3 at the end of the book).

Task 3: Drawing Kevin's family tree (and your own)

Drawing a family tree, also known as a genogram, is a good way to organise information about relationships in an easily accessible way and can help to 'break the ice' when starting to talk with a family, getting to know who is who within the family system (Task 1 above) and assisting with some of the previous tasks.

Try to include parents, grandparents, siblings, pets, etc., making it clear who lives in the household. The members of the household could be captured inside a line (circle, ellipse or any other shape to suit your family tree). In the family tree, male is represented by a square and female by a circle. It is common practice to write down the age of the person inside the square or the circle, with their name just below.

Therefore, a family tree can include details on gender, age and relationships, as well as an illness history. McGoldrick and Gerson (1985) offer a good description of how to draw a family tree.

After drawing the family tree, one could move on to family history of mental health problems (including addictions and history of abuse), occupation of family members, family relationships and social issues (such as neighbourhood, financial constraints, etc.).

Now would be a good time to draw first your family tree and then move on to drawing Kevin's family tree, based upon the information in the scenario (*see* Appendix 4 after completing the task).

Task 4: Identifying and dealing with a deadlock

A deadlock can occur between the clinician and the patient, or between different members of the family. In our scenario it could happen between Kevin and his mother, or between any of them and the clinician.

> Chloe believes it is all down to Kevin's behaviour. She says, 'He should just pull himself together and grow up'. She thinks that Kevin always acts to get a reaction from people. She is not shocked at the self-harm because she also does it. Chloe believes that thoughts of harming others are Kevin's way to attract attention and manipulate others.
>
> Kevin does not think he has a problem, but is willing to volunteer any information if asked about it. He resents that his mother has always been so busy with his siblings. Clearly, Kevin and his mother have different goals for being here and they will both need to be asked questions and have the opportunity to raise concerns.

A deadlock will be marked by a sense of stagnation in which any advice from the clinician results in a lack of change in the patient, who would generally resort to a *Yes, but* . . . reply to any advance from the clinician (e.g. advice that the patient should take medication to get better or to prevent deterioration, or have a conversation about how others view him).

With regard to treatment adherence, as a result of the clinician's knowledge of disease and its management being assumed to be superior to the patient's, it is also assumed that the patient will automatically agree with the assessment and the treatment plan. With this frame of mind, it is easy to see how a deadlock can arise and, for instance, a patient with depression may take antidepressants only when feeling depressed, rather than regularly, 'forgetting' that the treatment may take weeks to have any effect, or Kevin might consider that self-harming is a normal way of coping with stress because he has seen his mother doing it.

In this situation, the clinician is likely to become more and more frustrated and the patient more and more rigid, or in the case of Chloe and Kevin, both of them could become entrenched in their beliefs that the problems lie somewhere else. Behind this, there may be a belief that treatment (any intervention, really) only makes a problem worse (*I know someone who got awful side effects or killed himself while taking these tablets* or *What is the point of talking about things with Mum, nothing ever changes . . .*).

To avoid the potential deadlock, the clinician should check whether the patient (and the relatives) understand/s the treatment goals (the role of the medication or of a family intervention), giving opportunities to ask questions.

Task 5: The issue of 'secrets' and how to talk about them

When dealing with families, the issue of suppressed information can lead to difficulties. Secrecy-related problems are a recurrent feature of clinical management and can arise between clinicians and patients, patients and their families, and amongst clinicians.

> Chloe is aware that Kevin went through a 'goth' phase and that he has lacerated his forearms on occasions, but she is not aware that he visits suicide websites and that he has accessed pornographic websites involving children.

A boy treated by CAMHS for depression might also take ecstasy and smoke cannabis or access pornography, suicide or 'tips how to be a successful anorexic' websites but does not wish this shared with his family, or information might be known within a circle of relationships, but might be withheld from others.

So, how could we manage secrets?

➤ First of all, we should establish if a secret exists at all (drug use, issues around sexuality, experiences of abuse, and self-harm are common themes).

➤ If so, are there any legal concerns? (Risk to self or others, accessing pornographic websites involving minors, etc.).

➤ Third, consider sharing the dilemma with the clinical team and in supervision, weighing the advantages and disadvantages of keeping the secret.

➤ Fourth, ask hypothetical questions in a non-confrontational manner to help people imagine the consequences and consider ideas they might otherwise fear to address. An example of this would be:
Clinician: *Imagine your mum knows about you looking at the Internet with children . . .*

➤ Fifth, without disclosing the confidential information, discuss hypothetical possibilities, for instance, asking Chloe, *What does Kevin's reluctance to talk about his problems say to you?* whilst also establishing with the patient (Kevin in our scenario) who can be told about the secret.

Therefore, how could we reduce the chance of getting drawn into difficult dynamics and maximise the chances of achieving a shared understanding?

➤ Acknowledge the support of all parties/persons/agencies trying to help.
➤ Give them time to raise issues and concerns.
➤ Before giving information to others, try to give it first to the patient.
➤ Write up a summary in the notes of important discussions with relatives/other agencies. This will help other clinicians.
➤ Enlist the family to assist with treatment adherence, without making assumptions as to who the patient regards as family.
➤ Work through secrets, rather than ignoring them.
➤ Use hypothetical questions as a way to help overcome a deadlock.

Experience working with families and relatives in mental health is of great importance here. Nevertheless, the skills you are gaining are transferable to most other clinical settings.

OSCE practice task 6

Focusing on the chapter's scenario and spending only 5 minutes, identify, through formulated questioning, who is important in Kevin's family, who Kevin considers as family and how he views the relationships with them.

OSCE practice task 7

Utilising only 5 minutes, formulate at least 10 questions (two for each section) that you could be asking to take a psychological history of Kevin, covering school and educational aspects, hobbies and activities, drug and alcohol use, sexuality and self-harm and issues of safety. You might need to infer some of the details that are not provided in the scenario. Use Appendix 3 at the end of this book as an aide-memoire.

OSCE practice task 8

Draw a family tree of the case described in this chapter's scenario.

OSCE practice task 9

List five possible deadlocks when speaking with Kevin and Chloe.

OSCE practice task 10

Identify five potential secrets that could exist in Kevin's family, based on the information provided in the scenario.

REFERENCES

Christie D, Viner R. Adolescent development. *BMJ*. 2005; **330**(7486): 301–4.

Goldenring JM, Cohen E. Getting into adolescent heads. *Contemp Pediatr*. 1998; **5**(7): 75–80.

Goldenring JM, Rosen DS. Getting into adolescent heads: an essential update. *Contemp Pediatr*. 2004; **21**(1): 64–90.

Kurtz SM, Silverman JD, Draper J. *Teaching and Learning Communication Skills in Medicine*. 2nd ed. Oxford: Radcliffe; 2005.

McGoldrick M, Gerson R. *Genograms in Family Assessment*. 1st ed. New York, NY: WW Norton; 1985.

FURTHER READING

Belzer EJ. *Skills Training in Communication and Related Topics. Part I: Dealing with conflict and change*. Oxford: Radcliffe; 2009.

Hinz C. *Communicating with Your Patients: skills for building rapport*. Chicago, IL: American Medical Association; 1999.

Jacobson JL, Jacobson AM. *Psychiatric Secrets*. 2nd ed. Philadelphia, PA: Hanley & Belfus; 2001.

Levetown M. Communicating with children and families: from everyday interactions to skill in conveying distressing information. *Pediatrics*. 2008; **121**: 1441–60.

Lloyd M, Bor R. *Communication Skills for Medicine*. Edinburgh: Churchill Livingstone; 2004.

Mengel MB. *Introduction to Clinical Skills: a patient-centered textbook*. 1st ed. New York, NY: Kluwer Academic/Plenum; 1996.

Pendleton D, Schofield T, Tate P, *et al*. *The Consultation: developing doctor-patient communication*. Oxford: Oxford University Press; 2003.

Smith R. *Patient-Centred Interviewing: an evidence based method*. 1st ed. Phildelphia, PA: Lippincott, Williams & Wilkins; 2002.

CHAPTER 8

Assessment of mental capacity

Andrew Tarbuck and Roger Wesby

LEARNING OUTCOMES

- To know how to assess cognitive function, current level of ability and risk in a sensitive manner
- To know when and how to use an informant
- To know the general principles regarding the assessment of mental capacity in all patients and specifically how to assess capacity in a patient with dementia in relation to making decisions regarding driving, living accommodation and accepting appropriate help

INTRODUCTION

All clinicians assess mental capacity many times each day. Often this is an automatic, subliminal process because the patient clearly follows the discussion, understands the information provided and is able to make valid decisions.

Sometimes you may suspect that your patient lacks capacity to make a particular decision. This is often because of cognitive impairment due to dementia or delirium, which are conditions commonly encountered in older people, and very frequently in clinical practice. For example, the average district general hospital of 500 beds will, at any point in time, have approximately:

➤ 330 patients aged over 65
➤ 102 with dementia
➤ 66 with delirium (Royal College of Psychiatrists, 2005).

The issue of reduced mental capacity will also be encountered in some patients with a learning disability or with serious mental illness.

TABLE 8.1 Skills for you to apply (using the Calgary–Cambridge Guides) to assess Mental Capacity

Skills from the CC guides	*Applying these skills with greater depth, intention and intensity*
Initiation	
Develop rapport	Special consideration needs to be given to people who have medical, neurological or sensory problems that may interfere with communication (e.g. dysphasia following CVA, dysarthria and hypophonia in Parkinson's disease, deafness or visual impairment). Many older patients are seen with a relative or other caregiver: here rapport needs to be carefully developed with all parties.
Screen	The clinician needs to remember that screening and prioritisation are particularly important with older people because of the potential presence of multiple problems or disabilities over time. Remember that: • the type and number of problems do not necessarily predict function • not all problems are current • not all need help • not all are on the patient's agenda.
Listen attentively	Gauging the patient's emotional state early and throughout the interview is very important when consulting with the elderly: both anxiety and depression are common in the elderly and may not present overtly.
Gathering information	
Ask clarifying questions *Time frame* *Summarise*	Often with older patients, the clinician listens to a complex narrative, with large amounts of seemingly elusive data; here the skills of clarification, assessing time frame, summarising and checking become very important, for example explicitly requesting that the patient explain their problem from when it began up to the present or over a particular time period can be helpful.
Pick up cues	The patient may be embarrassed or scared by their problem and this can lead to a reluctance to admit to memory problems for fear of being 'put away' or because of the stigma of a diagnosis such as dementia or Alzheimer's disease. The expectations and attitudes of older people towards health & social services (e.g. that help from social services is 'charity' which is demeaning) can also make people reluctant to ask for help. Picking up, checking out and responding to non-verbal or verbal cues is therefore particularly important.
Use language appropriately	Clear, simple language is required if the patient is confused, disorientated, upset or has speech or hearing difficulties. Begin by checking out assumptions about what is contributing to the communication difficulties. Is pain or side effects of medication a factor? Is jargon or the language in which you are speaking a problem? When a patient is dysarthric or deaf, check understanding and whether the patient would find it easier to communicate via the written word. Check if the patient uses hearing aids, and if so, whether they are in place and in working order.

Skills from the CC guides	*Applying these skills with greater depth, intention and intensity*
Discover the patient's perspective	The patient's perspective is all important here – the effect that the condition has on the patient's life often predicts the patient's expectations or follow-through regarding treatment and needs to be carefully taken into consideration. Take into account the role of the patient's family (e.g. what help is the older person receiving from their family and what help is the older person providing to younger generations, for example childcare?).

Building the relationship

Demonstrate appropriate non-verbal behaviour	Show patience and give sufficient time: going at the patient's pace is vital.
Demonstrate sensitivity, empathy, acceptance and support	Older patients and their significant others may need a great deal of emotional as well as practical support. Attempting to appreciate the predicament the patient is in may help you to understand what at first sight is awkward or unusual behaviour. Consider the patient's past life, current situation and plans or concerns regarding the future (e.g. the patient was brought up in a children's home and has a consequent dread of institutions). The response to such issues should be empathic and respectful; offer practical help and support. Help patients and families navigate the complexities of health and social care agencies.

Structuring the interview

Summarise *Signpost*	Using these two skills in tandem may be particularly useful with older patients, particularly those who have hearing difficulties and loss of memory. Elderly patients can become lost in their own complex narrative and need help in structuring their own account: summarising and signposting therefore helps both patient and clinician. Structuring the consultation allows the clinician to check out questions or plans with carers as well as the patient: *I know that you find it hard to get out to do the shopping now . . . Can I just check with your daughter a moment . . . Where do you live?* A memory test can be a useful tool of assessment with elderly patients; this needs to be signposted carefully to avoid embarrassment or anger.

Explanation and planning

Chunk and check	Chunk and check, using clear language free from jargon.
Use diagrams	Using diagrams and written instructions, particularly in relation to medication, is helpful for those with memory loss and for their caregivers.

As a clinician, the commonest mental capacity issue is whether the patient can give valid consent or refusal to a proposed treatment. However, you may also be asked for opinions regarding a patient's capacity to undertake a wide variety of decisions and tasks, such as: to agree to hospital admission or take their own discharge, to manage their finances, to make a valid will or Lasting Power of Attorney, to drive a vehicle and to accept or refuse practical support and help at home.

SKILLS FOR YOU TO APPLY

Older people constitute a rapidly increasing sector of the population and are major users of health services. Good communication skills with older people are, therefore, crucial. Many older people also have cognitive impairment and this can present a significant challenge for both clinician and patient. Early identification of cognitive difficulty (e.g. concentration, memory or language) may allow you to compensate for or 'work around' the problems.

The Calgary–Cambridge (CC) model does provide some guidance on particular communication skills that may be helpful in working with this group of patients. These are summarised in Table 8.1 on pages 84–85 (adapted from Silverman *et al.*, 2005).

There is clear evidence from a large number of studies that good communication between clinicians and older patients is linked with positive health outcomes (Stewart *et al.*, 2000). Key factors include:

➤ gaining agreement between clinician and patient regarding the expectations of the interview
➤ encouraging the patient to ask questions and participate actively
➤ sensitive and timely information giving
➤ provision of 'take home' written information
➤ making the discussion relevant to the patient's situation
➤ demonstrating a caring attitude by listening and showing empathy.

Scenario

Elizabeth Johnson has come with her mother, Marjorie Williams (aged 79) to the interview.

Mrs Williams normally lives with her husband (Bert), but he has recently been admitted to hospital and is being placed into nursing home care. Following his admission to hospital, Mrs Williams has been muddled, has had difficulty in cooking and managing household tasks. There have been recent problems with her wandering away from home, looking for Bert. She has very little recollection of these events and has limited insight into her problems.

Mrs Johnson had noticed increasing forgetfulness in her mother for perhaps 2–3 years. However, until her father was admitted to hospital, she had not really appreciated the severity of her mother's problems. It has now become apparent that Bert had been 'covering up' for Marjorie and had very gradually taken over most household tasks. Bert has told Elizabeth that Marjorie has gradually become more repetitive and forgetful. Bert was going shopping with Marjorie (she was driving as he is partially sighted), but he had to tell her which way to go. She could not find the supermarket if he did not give her instructions. Bert has also told Elizabeth that there have been several 'close shaves' (e.g. she has gone through red traffic lights, mounted the kerb on three or four occasions and has bumped into another car whilst parking). He has also said that Marjorie has become rather irritable towards him, that she no longer reads the newspaper or watches TV and instead wanders about the house in an aimless fashion or talks about events from many years ago.

HOW TO DO IT

The key tasks are:

1 Develop skills in communicating with cognitively impaired patients.
2 Learn how to work with both a patient and an informant (a triadic consultation).
3 Make an assessment of current level of practical ability and risks in someone with cognitive impairment.
4 Know how to assess cognitive function in a sensitive manner.
5 Learn how to make simple capacity assessments in patients with dementia.

Task 1: Communicating with cognitively impaired patients

If you know that a patient has cognitive impairment, then it is possible to prepare in advance for the interview (e.g. by obtaining old case notes, speaking with other professionals involved and arranging to have a relative or carer present.)

Sometimes, the presence of cognitive impairment may only be suspected part-way through an interview. Under these circumstances, guide the interview into an assessment of cognitive function. Identifying cognitive impairment will keep you from sinking into a morass of non-information.

Try to develop a rapport with the patient and understand things from their perspective. It can be helpful to have a brief 'social chat' first (e.g. about their journey to the hospital or the weather). If the patient is suspicious, defensive or unwilling to talk, try spending the first part of the interview on 'safe' or 'emotionally neutral' topics (such as their background and social history). Leave potentially threatening or contentious issues (such as a discussion about driving) until later in the interview.

Task 2: Working with a patient and an informant

When working with patients who have (or are suspected to have) cognitive impairment, it is vital to obtain a collateral history from someone who knows the patient well. This is because people with cognitive impairment often lack insight into the nature, extent and degree of their problems and the practical consequences.

There are several ways of working with a patient and informant. These include:

1 conducting the interview jointly with both patient and informant at the same time (i.e. a triadic consultation)
2 separating patient and informant and interviewing both independently
3 conducting totally separate interviews with the patient and with the inform-ant (at different times in different locations, possibly even conducting the informant interview by telephone)
4 a combination of the above.

Don't say:

> *Right, Mrs Williams, you just wait there and I'll discuss things with your daughter in the next room and decide if you are safe to remain at home.*

The approach undertaken will depend on the availability of an informant (e.g. a relative who works may only be contactable by telephone), the nature of the relationship between patient and informant, and the wishes of both parties. Sometimes an informant may clearly indicate that there is additional information they wish to give to the clinician 'but not in front of my mother'. Occasionally a triadic consultation can become too contentious or disputed (e.g. if the patient disagrees vehemently with the carer's viewpoint), in which case it may be neces-sary to conduct the interviews separately.

If possible, try to adopt strategy 1 (above). The patient has support from a familiar person and all information is given 'in the open', which avoids patients' concerns that 'things are being said behind my back'. Undertaking the interview in this way clearly illustrates how much insight the patient has into their situation and problems. It is, however, necessary to manage the interview well. Signpost clearly, make sure that both patient and informant have the opportunity to put forward their views and ensure that a balance is maintained between both par-ties. Although most relatives have the best interests of the patient at heart, an informant's views may be coloured by other factors (e.g. unrealistic avoidance of all risks, inability/unwillingness to continue in the caring role or financial motives).

Try this instead:

Clinician: *Good morning. I'm* (insert name and profession) *and I've come to see you both today to have a chat about how things are going and see if there is anything I can do to help. You must be Mrs Williams.*

Patient: *That's right.*

Informant: *And I'm her daughter, Elizabeth.*

Clinician: *I'm very pleased to meet you. Your daughter asked if we could all meet up today because, since your husband has gone into hospital, she has noticed that you seem to be having some difficulties with your memory.*

Patient: *Well, I'm worried sick about Bert! That's all it is.*

Clinician: *Of course you are, and you are right; stress can cause difficulties with concentrating and remembering things. However, there are lots of reasons why people may have memory difficulties and I would like to find out more about what is happening at present, because I may be able to offer you some help or treatment. I want to ask you both some questions to find out how your memory has been recently and about how you have been managing at home. Perhaps I could start by asking you some questions, Mrs Williams? Then I will ask your daughter for her thoughts a little later on. Would that be all right?*

Task 3: Assessment of current level of ability and risks

Patients with cognitive impairment often lack insight and may be unaware that they are not coping well or need help. Sometimes this can reach the point where they present a risk to themselves or others. A detailed collateral history from an informant who knows the patient and their current circumstances well (e.g. a relative, carer, social worker) is very important in exploring these issues. It will provide some 'evidence' of how the person with cognitive impairment is functioning and provides some measure of 'objective risk'.

In relation to assessing someone's capacity to make a particular decision or undertake a particular task, then one would be particularly interested in the risks related to that task or decision and to the patient's level of insight. It will also be essential to find out if the patient agrees with the 'objective risks' and will accept any necessary measures to mitigate the risk.

As regards capacity to be able to remain at home safely, the areas of interest are widespread and include:

➤ self-care (washing, dressing, continence, eating and drinking)
➤ shopping, food preparation, laundry and cleaning the house
➤ managing finances (getting pension, paying bills, losing money)
➤ wandering or getting lost
➤ fire or flood (leaving gas on or taps running, smoking habits)
➤ aggression
➤ help being provided and willingness to accept it.

It is also useful to ask about areas of function that are well preserved and about activities that the person is coping with successfully.

Don't say:

> *Mrs Williams, I need to find out if you are safe to be at home. Let me ask you, Mrs Johnson; has your mother been doing anything dangerous at home?*

Try this instead:

> Clinician: *Mrs Williams, could I ask you how you have been managing with getting food and meals recently?*
>
> Patient: *Oh, there's no problem there! I'm a good cook. I used to work as a cook at the local school. I can still cook a good roast dinner with all the trimmings.*
>
> Clinician: *Are you still cooking regularly now that your husband is in hospital? People often find they can't really be bothered to cook a meal for one.*
>
> Patient: *Well, sometimes . . . But I still cook regularly for myself; sausage and mash, homemade soup, shepherd's pie . . .*
>
> Clinician: *Can I ask your daughter how she feels the cooking is going?*
>
> Informant: *Well, Mum's right, she was an excellent cook. However, she hasn't been doing nearly as much cooking recently. Since Dad has been in hospital she's been living on cakes and biscuits and the food I bought her has gone off in the fridge.*

It is not always appropriate to rely solely on information from informants and sometimes it will be helpful to obtain more direct evidence of functional abilities, for example, via an occupational therapy assessment.

Task 4: Cognitive assessment

The assessment of cognitive function is an important part of capacity assessment (although it does not, by itself, provide sufficient evidence to decide whether or not a person has or lacks capacity to make a particular decision). When thinking about cognitive assessment in this context, it is helpful to 'go back to first principles' and consider why one is assessing various aspects of cognitive function. For example:

➤ Language and comprehension – can the patient understand the information given to them and communicate their decisions effectively?

➤ Attention and concentration – can they focus on the task?

➤ Memory – can they retain the information long enough to come to a decision?

➤ Frontal-executive function – can they believe the information given to them and can they make reasoned judgements?

In clinical practice, this is often undertaken using an assessment tool such as the Abbreviated Mental Test Score (Hodkinson, 1972), the Mini-Mental State Examination (MMSE) (Folstein *et al.*, 1975) or the revised Addenbrooke's Cognitive Examination (Hodges, 2007). The MMSE is the most widely used test, although it should be recognised that it does not examine all areas of cognitive function (e.g. frontal-executive function) and sometimes additional tests are needed.

Poor performance on cognitive tests is not diagnostic of dementia. All that a low score demonstrates is that the person is having difficulty in answering the questions! This could be for a variety of reasons, including dementia, delirium, severe depression, dysphasia, lack of fluency in English, etc. As with any condition, the diagnosis of dementia should be made on the basis of a good history (from an informant as well as the patient), examination (physical and mental state examination) and any relevant investigations.

Tips on cognitive assessment

➤ Some patients can feel threatened and belittled by such assessments. Hence try to make it as 'matter of fact' as possible and employ strategies to help the person feel at ease. This includes avoiding telling them that they have got something 'wrong' and rescuing them from questions with which they are having difficulty. Calling it a 'quiz' sounds less imposing.

➤ Remember that stress/anxiety will diminish cognitive performance. Building a *good rapport* and helping the patient relax will improve their performance; allowing them to become flustered may mean the test has to be abandoned.

➤ Be flexible about the timing of the cognitive assessment during the interview. Early testing (*after* a therapeutic alliance has been formed) can help determine the reliability of responses to questions of fact (e.g. about family members or home circumstances). Test cognitive function *before* discussing contentious issues like driving or safety to remain at home.

➤ Try to use as few words as possible during the process. However (and this is the art) do add one or two 'conversational' phrases to help the patient feel that they are not being interrogated. Take into consideration any hearing difficulty. If a question is not heard, repeat using the same words (speaking slowly, clearly and loudly). Ensure that the patient is wearing their hearing aid or glasses.

➤ Watch for *cues* indicating that your patient is losing interest or getting irritated. Be prepared to complete the examination at a later date if necessary.

➤ Be sensitive about giving feedback. However, if the patient realises they have had difficulty with some test items, this can provide a useful introduction to starting a discussion regarding their cognitive problems.

Don't say:

> Clinician: *Right, Mrs Williams. I'm going to test your cognitive abilities now. What year is it?*
> Patient: *Oh, I don't know. I never use it. Is it 1995?*
> Clinician: *No, it's 2011.*

Try this instead:

> Clinician: *I would now like to test your memory with a quiz. These are routine questions I ask everyone. Some of the questions are a bit daft but please put up with them! Your daughter/son mustn't help with the answers.*
> Patient: *Oh, I don't know, what happens if I get it all wrong?*
> Clinician: *Try not to worry. There is no 'pass' or 'fail'. I'm asking these questions to find out how well your memory is working so that I will know how best to help.*
> Patient: *Alright.*
> Clinician: *What year is it?*
> Patient: *Oh, I don't know. I never use it. Is it 1995?*
> Clinician: *OK. What about the season?*

Task 5: Capacity assessment

Capacity assessment is not a 'blanket process'. Capacity assessments look at the capacity of an individual to undertake a particular activity/task at a particular point in time. Legally, adults are presumed to have capacity unless proven otherwise. An unwise decision does not of itself indicate lack of capacity.

In England and Wales, the Mental Capacity Act provides a legal framework to guide many of the decisions relating to capacity assessment and the management of those lacking capacity. There is similar legislation in Scotland. Some tasks have clear criteria (laid down in statute or case law) that need to be fulfilled in order for the patient to have capacity (for example, the capacity to make a will). Other tasks have no specific legal criteria and a decision has to be made on the basis of common sense and the best evidence available (e.g. does someone have the capacity to manage their finances or to decide where they should live?).

In general, the more 'serious or significant' the decision, the greater the degree of capacity required.

Mental capacity is assessed using a two-stage process:

1 Is there an impairment of, or disturbance in the functioning of, the person's mind or brain?

2   Is the impairment or disturbance sufficient that the person lacks the capacity to make that particular decision? This is addressed using the 'functional test' of capacity (see below).

Both of the above need to be demonstrated in order to say that someone lacks capacity. Just because a person has a condition that impairs brain function (e.g. dementia) does *not* automatically mean that they lack capacity.

The 'functional test' of capacity covers four areas. In order to have capacity, it is necessary to:

➤ understand what decision has to be made
➤ understand and assess the information relating to the decision (e.g. benefits, risks, alternatives) and understand the consequences of these possible choices
➤ retain the information long enough to 'weigh the information in the balance' and make an effective decision
➤ communicate this decision.

If a person is unable to do *any one* of these things, then they lack capacity.

It is important that the clinician makes all efforts to optimise communication with the patient (e.g. that things have been explained in sufficiently simple terms for the patient to understand).

Assessment of capacity to decide where one should live

There are no clear criteria or legal test cases and judgement is based on clinical assessment. Factors to consider include:

➤ What is the cause and severity of the cognitive impairment?
➤ Does the person know where they live (current address) and their current living circumstances (who is at home, what help they currently receive)?
➤ Is the person aware of the nature and degree of their problems and the potential risks involved in being at home?
➤ How well are they currently managing at home?
➤ Is there evidence of current risks and how severe are they?
➤ Are they able to understand information about their problems and the type and amount of help they need?
➤ Are they willing to accept appropriate help or consider appropriate alternatives?
➤ Are they being realistic and consistent in what they say?

Assessment of capacity to drive

In the UK the Driver Vehicle Licensing Authority (DVLA) publishes criteria regarding fitness to drive in various medical conditions in their document

At a Glance Guide to the Current Medical Standards of Fitness to Drive (www.dft. gov.uk/dvla/medical/ataglance.aspx).

With regard to dementia, they acknowledge that the assessment of capacity to drive may be difficult and that in some cases a formal driving assessment may be required. Significant impairment of short-term memory, orientation, insight, judgement or attention would almost certainly preclude driving. In early dementia, where sufficient skills are retained and progression is slow, DVLA may issue a licence on an annual basis. A decision regarding fitness to drive is usually based on medical reports.

Don't say:

Clinician: *I need to assess if you are still safe to drive, Mrs Williams.*
Patient: *Of course I am! I've been driving for over 30 years and never had an accident. There aren't any problems there!*
Clinician: *OK then, that's fine.*

Try this instead:

Clinician: *Do you drive a car, Mrs Williams?*
Patient: *Yes! I've been driving for over 30 years and never had an accident. There aren't any problems there!*
Clinician: *Alright, but I would also like to ask your daughter for her thoughts. Mrs Johnson, how do you think your mother's driving is at present?*
Informant: *I am very worried about her driving. Dad has told me that she has had a few 'close shaves' recently. She has gone through several red lights and last month she bashed into another car at the supermarket.*

OSCE practice task 11

You have been asked to see Mrs Marjorie Williams (79) and her daughter (Mrs Johnson) on the orthopaedic ward.

Mrs Williams fell at home 3 weeks ago, sustaining a fractured left neck of femur. She can now walk with a frame, but since surgery she has been more muddled than previously. Mrs Williams is insistent on returning home.

A home assessment with the occupational therapist and physiotherapist revealed the following:

- She cannot manage stairs (bathroom, toilet and bedroom are upstairs).
- To return home safely, they advise that a commode and bed would need to be placed downstairs and she would require help with washing, dressing, preparing meals and emptying the commode.

Your task is to interview Mrs Williams and her daughter and make an assessment of her capacity to decide about returning home.

Your time is limited and any cognitive assessment should be brief. A 10-point Abbreviated Mental Test pro forma is available if you wish to use it.

In the last minute, you will discuss the case with the assessor.

You have 10 minutes for this station.

REFERENCES

Folstein MF, Folstein SE, McHugh PR. A practical method for grading the cognitive state of patients for the clinician. *J Psychiat Res.* 1975; **12**: 189–98.

Hodges JR. The Addenbrooke's cognitive examination – revised and supplementary test suggestions. In: Hodges JR. *Cognitive Assessment for Clinicians.* 2nd ed. Oxford: Oxford University Press; 2007. pp. 157–83.

Hodkinson, HM. Evaluation of a mental test score for assessment of mental impairment in the elderly. *Age Ageing.* 1972; **1**: 233–8.

Royal College of Psychiatrists. *Who Cares Wins. Improving the outcome for older people admitted to the general hospital: guidelines for the development of liaison mental health services for older people. A report of a working group for the Faculty of Old Age Psychiatry.* London: Royal College of Psychiatrists; 2005.

Silverman J, Kurtz S, Draper J. *Skills for Communicating with Patients.* 2nd ed. Oxford: Radcliffe; 2005.

Stewart M, Meredith l, Brown JB, *et al.* The influence of older patient-physician communication on health and health-related outcomes. *Clin Geriatr Med.* 2000; **16** (1): 25–36. www.dft.gov.uk/dvla/medical/ataglance.aspx

FURTHER READING

British Medical Association, Law Society. *Assessment of Mental Capacity: a practical guide for doctors and lawyers.* 3rd ed. London: Law Society; 2010.

Hodges JR. *Cognitive Assessment for Clinicians.* 2nd ed. Oxford: Oxford University Press; 2007.

The Stationery Office. *Mental Capacity Act 2005: code of practice.* London: The Stationery Office; 2007.

CHAPTER 9

Dealing with emotions

Roger Wesby, Xavier Coll and Andrew Tarbuck

LEARNING OUTCOMES

- To understand the general principles of dealing with emotions in the consultation and thereby be able to interview skilfully and sensitively patients who are overtly emotional
- To have strategies for dealing with patients in more extreme emotional states
- To recognise the importance of the clinician's own inner feelings (intuition/countertransference) in the consultation process

INTRODUCTION

Emotions are present during every patient-clinician interaction and nowhere more so than in mental health consultations. They help or hinder the consultation process depending upon their nature and degree. This chapter looks at the principles of dealing with emotions and considers in more detail the skills needed to deal with distress and anger as well as strategies for dealing with more extreme emotions of rage and severe agitation. Possible consequences of the emotions felt by the clinician are also explored.

DEALING WITH EMOTIONS: GENERAL PRINCIPLES

1 Emotions are present in every consultation: from the more commonly considered, such as anxiety, anger and sadness, to the less frequently identified, such as shame.

2 Most patients attend a consultation because of concern about something; in other words, anxiety is usually present. It can be helpful to think of all

emotions being secondary: discovery of possible causal factors helps the clinician to develop understanding that in turn contributes to the development of empathy.

3 Emotions can both help and hinder the consultation process. On the one hand, they can drive the patient to seek help and facilitate the assessment process. On the other hand, emotions can preoccupy the patient and impact negatively on the consultation process by causing the patient to fail to engage with the clinician, thereby making it more difficult for the clinician to develop rapport with the patient.

4 Patients will differ in the degree to which they reveal any particular emotion. It may simply be not verbalised or be deeply hidden, resulting in the clinician having to pick up subtle body and verbal cues by employing what is described as 'active listening' (see below).

5 Most emotional patients benefit from the clinician conveying an empathetic response. Empathy – feeling on the same wavelength – can be achieved both by active listening and by facilitating the patient to express themselves through providing a feeling of trust and safety that the psychoanalyst Wilfred Bion described as 'containment' (Bion, 1962). This is achieved not only by the manner of the clinician but also by the environment: ensuring that the consulting room is as comfortable and free from interruptions as possible, for example by switching off mobile phones.

6 Expression of certain emotions, particularly distress, occurs because the patient feels secure enough to share their feelings with the clinician. Even expression of ordinary anger suggests that the patient feels confident that the clinician will not retaliate. Expression of such emotions, therefore, is a very direct and honest communication by the patient.

7 During heightened emotional states, spoken language may be difficult for patients both to verbalise and to understand. Research has shown that verbal areas of the brain can shut down during extremes of emotion (van der Kolk, 2004). The body language and tone of voice of the clinician become much more important during such times. Your patient is hurting emotionally: soothe them with the tone of your voice and respond in short sentences, simple vocabulary or utterances such as 'um' that convey that you are listening and are there with them.

8 Certain patient groups, particularly those with an early life history of abuse or maltreatment, can have more complex expression of emotions. Patients with emotionally unstable and so-called borderline personality disorder continue to use primitive defence mechanisms, such as projection, thereby enabling them to rid themselves of feelings by projecting them into others: they 'get under our skin'. Also, some such patients have difficulty putting words to their feelings (alexithymia) or even feeling the emotion. Powerful

emotions that are not felt psychologically can get enacted or 'acted out': the patient *does* something rather than feel the emotion, think about it and work it through.

9 Clinicians will also experience emotions in response to their patients (countertransference). The 'active listening' for cues should extend to the clinician themself: being watchful of their own inner feelings. Countertransference is particularly useful in situations where the patient's behaviour does not tally with the emotion being felt by the clinician. This is vital if there are feelings of threat or danger that enable the clinician to consider appropriate courses of action. It is also important for clinicians to be aware of how much their feelings are influencing their management of the patient: clinicians can also 'act out' if they are not aware of their feelings (Winnicott, 1949).

10 Whether or not the clinician should encourage expression and ventilation of an emotion depends upon several factors, such as the type of emotion. Anger is best 'managed' rather than being stoked up. Dealing with such emotions as distress depends upon such things as how well the clinician knows the patient, whether the patient is to be seen again and how much time is available before the end of the session. Clinicians vary in their ability to tolerate expressions of emotion from their patients and a common fear is one of unleashing uncontrollable feelings that the clinician will be unable to deal with.

SKILLS FOR YOU TO APPLY

Establishing initial rapport is crucial to the success of any interview with a patient in an aroused emotional state. Particular care should be taken with preparation of the consulting room environment and the manner of introduction.

Negotiating the agenda is particularly important. Try not to proceed with the interview until the agenda has been agreed upon. Notice the word 'negotiate': it should be based on both your and the patient's needs. More time may be needed to achieve this since distressed patients may not easily disclose what is on their minds initially. Watching for verbal and body cues will be necessary to pick up any covert content.

The agenda helps to **provide structure** to the interview – very important to an emotional patient who may be feeling vulnerable. Ongoing structure should be provided by signposting and summarising, and the sense of security can be enhanced further by '**active listening**'; that is, actively focusing attention to discern all information coming from the patient in words, body language and feelings. This can be facilitated by both non-verbal skills that convey an interest in the patient, such as eye contact, facial expression and body language, and verbal responses that encourage the patient to speak, including appropriate use of silence.

Finally, pay attention to **closing the session** well. A highly aroused patient will need time for the emotion to subside before feeling ready to face the outside world again. Paying as much attention to ending as beginning the interview makes it more likely that the patient will return to seek further help.

Scenario 1: Anger

Diane Webb, aged 45, teacher. She separated from her husband 6 years ago and has intermittent contact via the children. She has two children, the eldest, Robert (Bob), aged 22, is currently abroad. Her younger son, Edward (Eddy), aged 18, was living with her until recently and is studying philosophy at university.

Mrs Webb's background: a relatively happy childhood until her father lost his job and began drinking alcohol heavily in her teens. Both her parents are now dead. She can still vividly remember her father's rages following drinking alcohol when she was frightened that he might hurt her or her mother. As a result, she has always worried that her children may turn to alcohol, since she has read that a tendency to alcoholism is hereditary. Her parents never sought any help for her father's alcohol problem. They frequently talked of her grandmother being taken to the 'loony bin' where patients ('nutters') were treated appallingly and simply shut away. She continues to feel that any problem with mental health is shaming and she would never admit to having any 'weakness' like depression. In fact, she has been feeling significantly stressed out recently because of her stressful job. It would not cross her mind to seek help from her GP about her poor sleep.

Today's situation: Mrs Webb was telephoned at 4 a.m. this morning to be told that Eddy had been admitted to an acute psychiatric ward. Staff would give her no information over the telephone (Eddy has agreed to his mother being informed only of his admission), and she had left immediately from home and arrived at the hospital at about 6 a.m. It is now just after 9 a.m. and she has been waiting all this time for someone to give her information. She has been told that the duty doctor who has been working all night is unavailable because he is not on this hospital site. The nursing staff also seem to be too busy and have kept telling her that she must wait for the ward doctor. The nurses changed shifts at 7:30 a.m. and she had expected the ward doctor to arrive at this time.

Eddy: has been living in student digs. Mrs Webb sees him occasionally, but he has become more distant recently and coming home less often with his washing and for a meal. The last time she saw him, she thought he looked a bit scruffy and was a bit offhand with her. He did not seem to want to speak to her and she felt he was hiding something from her. She had wondered whether this was something to do with her ex-husband, Carl, with whom she has a rather volatile relationship. The boys have continued to see Carl. Carl has a very good job and is able to give the boys quite large sums of money that she disapproves of.

She has been particularly concerned recently about Eddy since she has been also wondering whether he might have been drinking or smoking cannabis or worse. This has been adding to her stress of late.

Ideas: Mrs Webb feels sure there has been a mistake here. Her son is not mentally ill and she plans to take him home immediately. He has not been looking after himself, not been eating properly and if he was to come home with her all will be well. Psychiatric hospitals are for nutters and no son of hers is going to stay in one.

Concerns: At the back of her mind, Mrs Webb does wonder whether he has been using alcohol or drugs, but she doesn't wish to admit this to anyone. Apart from her obvious concern for Eddy, who will be deeply distressed being in a psychiatric hospital, she is also very concerned about her work: this is a weekday, she has lessons booked all day and the head teacher (with whom she had an argument last week) is unsympathetic. She is already wondering what excuse she will give regarding her lateness. She intends to pick up her son and leave as soon as possible.

Dealing with anger

Mrs Webb (standing up, looking agitated): *At last! I've been waiting here since 6 a.m. No one will tell me what's happening. The nurses are avoiding me. My son's here in hospital and I want to take him home. I'm sick of being offered cups of tea! It's past 9 o'clock now and I should be at work. Just tell me how I can get my son out of here!*

How should the doctor respond to this?
Don't say:

Doctor (sitting down, looking annoyed, avoiding eye contact, getting out his notepad and writing on it): *Well, I'm here now. Let's get started because I haven't much time. I don't really know what's happened.*

As always, the task is to facilitate communication and in this case Mrs Webb's anger needs to subside to allow proper communication.

Recognise and acknowledge the emotion(s). In this scenario it may be obvious, but patients can present with mixed pictures. Anger is usually secondary to another feeling such as fear and/or, as in this scenario perhaps, shame.

Allow the patient to ventilate their feelings uninterrupted. This is not always easy! However attacking it may feel, remember that this is not a personal attack on you but that you represent 'the system'. It is not your fault that her son is in hospital. It is not your fault that she has had to wait to see you. Thinking like this helps to reduce any temptation to retaliate (a natural reaction in ordinary human interactions). In addition, Mrs Webb needs the doctor to be able to withstand her angry comments – to offer her a firm boundary against which she can rail. No, this may not feel comfortable, but it offers emotional containment.

Apologise, if appropriate, without accepting personal blame.

Try this instead:

> Doctor (looking concerned and unhurried, allowing patient to finish her outburst): *Mrs Webb? I'm Doctor Smith. I'm so sorry you've had to wait so long. Let's see how I can help you.*

Saying this does not imply that it is your fault; you are only sympathising with her. It is vital that you *look* sorry when you say this! It is also important to convey to the patient as accurately as possible that the feeling has been recognised. Angry feelings are often an attack and will be felt by you as such. It is usually helpful to show the patient that you have felt their anger by a facial expression that communicates 'ouch!' Remaining expressionless or, worse, smiling, will make matters worse.

> Doctor (looking solemn): *I can see that you're very angry. It must have been very frustrating not to have been given more information and to have been kept waiting for so long.*

Overtly acknowledging the patient's feelings helps to develop rapport. Watch for body cues to help determine when you can move the interview on, and, as always, negotiate an agenda. This is especially important if the anger is not subsiding: have you established all the reasons why Mrs Webb is so angry? This in itself will be therapeutic even though you do not have any answers for her: to be listened to, heard and understood are crucial.

What else not to say:

> Doctor, with little interest or care: *I know exactly how you're feeling.*
> Mrs Webb, more enraged: *What?!! How can you possibly know how I'm feeling?! How can you possibly know what it feels like to have a son locked away and be told that you can't see him?!*

Trying to convey to a patient that you have *some* understanding of their predicament is important and it is often better to put it in a more tentative fashion to help continue to build rapport. Such as:

Doctor: *I imagine that you must have felt pretty helpless stuck out here.*

There is rarely, however, a right or wrong thing to say and much will depend upon individual circumstances, especially the degree of rapport you have achieved. For example, to the sentence above the doctor could add: *You must be very worried about him*, which would flow naturally if the degree of rapport is good enough. If it is not, however, Mrs Webb could reply something like: *Don't tell me how I should be feeling!*

Responding appropriately and sensitively to such a situation, however, can both acknowledge the perceived blunder and develop rapport:

Doctor, looking concerned: *You're right. I can't know exactly how you're feeling. I'm just trying to understand how awful this situation must be for you at the moment.*

Once the anger has subsided sufficiently, the interview can continue along normal lines, bearing in mind that it may flare up again from time to time.

Scenario 2: Distress

Sarah Cheaney, aged 35, librarian; married to John for 15 years. Her only child, **Hannah**, aged 13, was killed tragically in a road traffic accident about 6 weeks ago. She has been referred to a psychiatrist by her GP who has become worried about her and wonders whether medication or psychotherapy may help.

Background: If asked casually, she had a 'happy' childhood; however, she was a lonely child of a mother who was indifferent to her, much too busy with her career in banking. She had no brothers or sisters. Her mother did all the functional things, but there was no 'wow factor'. As a teenager, she just got on with life and did not feel particularly different. She did reasonably well at school but lacked ambition. Her father was also busy with his work (a solicitor) and could be very loving at times, but these were very infrequent since he worked such long hours. She married only 6 months after meeting her husband, being already pregnant with Hannah. He was never the man of her dreams, but he had been a reasonably good husband and father, although he was increasingly absent with work commitments. Her life was transformed, however, with the birth of Hannah, who from the start was a perfect baby, full of vitality and happiness. Hannah had always wanted to be with her and had not wished to leave her to go to nursery or to school. Once settled, however, she was a very clever girl with many friends and is now (*she often thinks of her as alive still*) talented in both sport and music (Grade 2 piano). Even when Hannah grew older, she still preferred to spend time with her, rather than her friends; well, at least until about a year ago.

Hannah's death: Hannah was killed while riding her bicycle to her friend Naomi's house. A white van had hit her at speed at a crossroads. Mrs Cheaney has been told that the van driver was not at fault: he was not speeding and the lights were in his favour. She was killed instantly, a severe head injury. The incident is all a bit of a blur: police came round to her house, her husband identified the body and she arranged the funeral on autopilot. She barely remembers the funeral, where she showed little emotion and had become preoccupied with whether there would be enough food at the buffet at her home afterwards. Her main memory of the day is of the large groups of sobbing girls, friends of Hannah.

Since Hannah's death: Her husband has become increasingly withdrawn. He has barely spoken to her over the last fortnight. She tried to return to work, but was sent home after making several mistakes and being quite unable to concentrate. She has lost a stone in weight, not wishing to eat and knows that she has been worrying her GP. She is sleeping well with sleeping tablets. She feels blank and slightly detached rather than depressed. Suicide has never crossed her mind.

Behaviour: Mrs Cheaney is shut down with little emotional reactivity. She is passive and does not display anger outwardly. She has not spoken of her daughter's death since the funeral and she is on the verge of realising that Hannah is dead and will never come back. There is something that nobody yet knows which is tearing Mrs Cheaney apart, but she will be unable to disclose this unless she feels safe enough and can trust the doctor. If the interview situation feels safe enough, the anguish and sadness will begin to well up inside her for the first time. It is deeply painful. Hannah's lovely face keeps flashing into her mind.

Dealing with distress

Mrs Cheaney (no eye contact, wringing hands), after confirming her name, remains silent but struggling to speak for about 30 seconds before saying in a quiet voice: *I lost my daughter.*

Don't say:

> Doctor, looking unaffected by her distress: *Let's start with your medical history.*

Clearly, this is not the correct response but is an example of what might happen if the clinician becomes overwhelmed by the patient's feelings. Others include:

➤ premature reassurance (stopping them disclosing more)

➤ getting away from the uncomfortable subject matter by changing the subject or ending the interview early by prescribing medication or referring somewhere else

➤ asking more questions – taking control of the interview with a less collaborative approach, ignoring cues

➤ listening less – speaking faster with no pauses or silences

➤ feeling tired, bored or switched off

➤ becoming caught up in the emotion too strongly

➤ losing objectivity.

Similar skills for distress are used as in dealing with anger (above) and development of empathy is crucial: to get and stay on the person's wavelength. Your patient will be helped by feeling that you understand how she is feeling and what circumstances are contributing to this.

Identify the emotion: your patient must feel that you understand some of what she is feeling. Carefully check that you have got this right. Use active listening techniques: your intuition is usually a good judge here. Watch for any body and language cues.

Help your patient to communicate. This sounds obvious, but remember, an emotional patient may be feeling very vulnerable and need to feel safe before disclosing information. First impressions are crucial. Pay particular attention to initiating the session with regard to the physical surroundings, privacy and your body language. They will be wondering, *Can I trust this clinician?* Prepare yourself by clearing your mind of previous patients and problems and approach the patient openly and with an appropriate expression. Greetings, opening statements and identifying who you are should be clear and unhurried.

Try this instead:

Doctor, speaking slowly and softly, yet clearly, with unthreatening body language: *I'm so sorry. That's a terrible thing to have happened.*

It is vital to **negotiate the correct agenda**. The patient must feel that you understand their key concerns and these may not (and probably will not) be divulged immediately. How can the consultation progress with meaning if there are undisclosed agenda items and/or feelings?

Emotionally aroused patients may have difficulty in thinking and speaking: allow adequate time for their thoughts and feelings to be verbalised. This requires attention to pace, perhaps periods of silence and facilitating comments that may include simple words, phrases or utterances that help the patient feel that she is being heard and that you are listening.

Avoid using jargon. Think of the patient's emotional difficulties as a tangled ball of wool that must be gently teased out. Help the process along by using the same language and vocabulary as your patient, occasionally 'translating' if appropriate, for example naming what your patient keeps calling 'disappointment' as 'anger'.

The safer a patient is feeling with you, the more they can trust you. Adding structure to the interview conveys a sense of safety so summarising and signposting frequently are vital.

Should you touch the patient?

A very distressed patient may feel to you as if they need a hug. Whether you touch a patient depends upon such circumstances as their age (child, adult, older person), whether you are alone with them, how well you know them, location (clinic setting or patient's home) and whether or not there is any significant past history such as of abuse. Touching a patient is an action that can be a spontaneous gesture or a considered response. The latter is preferable: taking into consideration what you are feeling about the patient, why you are thinking that touching them is appropriate, whether touching them is appropriate at all, how you will touch them (hug or gentle contact with a shoulder) and what the advantages and disadvantages are of doing so.

Usually, patients can feel 'held' by our words, tone of voice and body language together with a strong feeling that we have them in mind. Together, these convey feelings that we are concerned, sympathetic and willing to help.

DEALING WITH EXTREMES OF EMOTION

Some patients under extreme stress or whose personality structure cannot deal with stress can present with extremes of emotion, such as agitation and extreme anger or rage. Principles of dealing with this are the same as in any interview – paying particular attention to cues, use of language and creating a safe containing environment.

Strategies for dealing with the enraged patient

Identify the emotion and degree of anger. It is helpful to differentiate between anger and rage. Anger is usually directed towards someone (you!) and, although uncomfortable, the patient can be reasoned with. Rage, on the other hand, is reminiscent of the blind rages of babies and is seen in patients with sensitive personality structures (narcissism, borderline). If this is the case, it is less easy to reason with the patient and they therefore may be unpredictable. Remember that their ability to understand spoken language may be temporarily impaired, so pay particular attention to your body language, vocabulary and tone of voice. Also, consider whether this is straightforward anger or whether there is also a degree of bitterness, hostility, vindictiveness or vengefulness. This helps reduce risk by identifying feelings that may be associated with a wish to hurt others.

Help yourself to feel safe by careful consideration of the physical environment, reading any available notes that may point to any acting-out behaviour in the past (violence). If you are feeling frightened, tactfully terminate the interview and start again once you have created a safer environment (e.g. with a co-worker). A very angry patient is feeling threatened in some way and is usually on high alert for signs of danger. It may not feel like it, but you may represent a threatening person: be cautious about the degree of eye contact (excessive eye contact can be threatening) and particularly cautious regarding touching the patient.

Remain constantly alert if the patient is behaving unpredictably. Enraged patients are more likely to 'act out' because they are unable to use more mature thinking and reasoning to defuse their state of mind. Constantly observe body language, tone of voice and eye contact, particularly if there is any change in these. Also observe your countertransference: trust any feelings of danger and act accordingly to reduce risk.

Remain calm and avoid looking/behaving in a threatening manner by using your body language, facial expression, position relative to the patient (i.e. not too close or far away), avoiding contradiction or argument and making sure the consultation is occurring in as safe an environment as possible.

A calm, confident demeanour will help to reassure your patient (although you may not be feeling like this inside!) as well as pointing out that they have choices (is not trapped).

The above suggestions aim to defuse the patient's degree of anger to a level when you can employ the strategies previously mentioned in this chapter. The situation will improve significantly once the patient feels safer and able to talk.

Skills for dealing with the very agitated or frightened patient

Very agitated patients can become overwhelmed by the emotion, possibly reliving some fearful experience. You cannot help them if you lose communication with them, i.e. they become dissociated from present reality. The following strategies are often helpful:

➤ Watch carefully for cues to determine the level of anxiety, such as rate of breathing, and whether it is escalating or not.

➤ To maintain rapport, you may need to speak more clearly, adjusting rate and volume of speech, possibly also saying their name or using body language to gain their attention.

➤ Help them to feel safe and unthreatened by your own body language – look calm and in control. You might also overtly give them permission not to answer questions with which they feel uncomfortable. If you sense that they may be reliving a frightening experience, remind them where they are and confirm that they are safe.

➤ Utilise such techniques as slow, controlled breathing.

➤ Do not explore very sensitive areas unless you have a clear purpose for knowing.

DEALING WITH OUR OWN EMOTIONS

The fact that we have feelings towards our patients during consultations (countertransference) has already been discussed. It is particularly important to identify feelings of anger or irritation with the patient that, if unidentified, may cause us to act out the feeling and react unfavourably in some way.

A small proportion of patients can stir up powerful emotions in us that remain with us after the patient has left. This can occur with so-called heartsink patients, (*see* Chapter 11) and in those patients whose life experiences may feel too close to our own. Being aware of and working with our own feelings towards patients can be exhausting work, particularly if such feelings remain with us for too long. Burnout can result or we may be tempted to employ unhealthy strategies, such as using excess alcohol or other substances.

Healthier strategies include discussing such feelings about patients with colleagues either informally (individually or in a group) or more formally in a Balint group. Once feelings are better understood, we can usually let them go and they are less likely to impact on patient management. Exercise, hobbies and friends and family are important sources of support and well-being. Finally, personal therapy can be invaluable to help us understand better ourselves and our emotional reactions to our patients.

OSCE practice task 12

You unexpectedly arrive 20 minutes late for a planned appointment with a 24-year-old man, Mr Jason Beck, whom you have seen twice previously, when you had seemed to get on very well. He is returning to discuss his response to prescribed medication for his anxiety and depression associated with the breakdown of a long-term relationship. You had discovered at his last visit that he had been adopted aged 3 years.

Mr Beck (standing up and looking flushed): *You're late! I've been here half an hour! What's the point of turning up if you can't be bothered to come!*

OSCE tasks

1 How would you respond to Mr Beck?
2 What skills should you employ to help reduce the intensity of Mr Beck's anger?

3 What could you do or say to make Mr Beck *more* angry?

4 What factors (past and present) might be fuelling Mr Beck's anger?

5 Mr Beck becomes much angrier, causing you to feel alarmed. How would you react to this?

REFERENCES

Bion WR. *Learning from Experience.* London: Heinemann; 1962. Chapter 27.

Lloyd M, Bor R. *Communication Skills for Medicine.* 3rd ed. New York, NY: Churchill Livingstone; 2009. Chapter 11.

Platt FW, Gordon GH. *Field Guide to the Difficult Patient Interview.* 2nd ed. Philadelphia, PA: Lippincott Williams and Wilkins; 2004. Chapter 9.

Van der Kolk BA. Psychobiology of posttraumatic stress disorder. In: Panksepp J, editor. *Textbook of Biological Psychiatry.* Hoboken, NJ: Wiley-Liss; 2004.

Winnicott D. Hate in the countertransference. *Int J Psychoanal.* 1949; **30**: 69–74.

FURTHER READING

Balint M. *The Doctor, His Patient and the Illness.* New York, NY: International Universities Press; 1957.

Cole S, Bird J. *The Medical Interview: the three-function approach.* St Louis, MO: Mosby; 2000.

Kurtz S, Silverman J, Draper J. *Teaching and Learning Communication Skills in Medicine.* 2nd ed. Oxford: Radcliffe; 2005.

Maguire P, Pitceathly C. Managing the difficult consultation. *Clin Med.* 2003; **3**(6): 532–7.

Silverman J, Kurtz S, Draper J. *Skills for Communicating with Patients.* 2nd ed. Oxford: Radcliffe; 2005.

CHAPTER 10

Breaking bad news in mental health

Xavier Coll and Sarah Maxwell

LEARNING OUTCOMES

- Incorporate the general skills of giving information and shared decision making into the structure of the psychiatric interview to explore difficulties with breaking bad news
- Describe the process of giving bad news

INTRODUCTION

Communicating bad news to a patient well is not an optional skill; it is an essential component of professional practice.

Breaking bad news in mental health is one of a clinician's most difficult duties, yet training typically offers little formal preparation for this daunting task. Without proper training, the discomfort and uncertainty associated with breaking bad news may lead clinicians to emotionally disengage from patients.

Patients generally desire frank and empathetic disclosure of a diagnosis or other bad news. Focused training in communication skills techniques to facilitate breaking bad news has been demonstrated to improve patient satisfaction and physician comfort.

The question of delivering 'bad' diagnostic news in psychiatry has generally been focused on dementia rather than functional psychiatric disorders and their effects. However, living with any serious psychiatric disorder and its consequences can mean losses in many areas of life, and could result in a bereavement reaction or even depression. As clinicians giving patients news of diagnosis or prognosis in psychiatry, we need to be aware of this and potentially intervene to support patients.

In addition to the potential loss of well-being, hope and health, the news may have an effect on relationships, change family roles (a partner becoming a carer, etc.), and bring about social stigma.

Clinicians sometimes avoid dealing with patients' emotional reactions to bad news, and so avoid providing a clear diagnosis for fear that patients or carers will be distressed. Patients may respond with denial and shock, which can make providing lengthy explanations difficult, and information may need to be given in small doses over a period of time.

In psychiatry, denial can also represent a lack of insight into a patient's condition, as many people with psychiatric illnesses do not accept that they are unwell. In these circumstances, ensuring that carers are available and also given appropriate information becomes essential.

Communicating bad news can be stressful for clinicians. Evidence suggests the bearer of bad news experiences strong emotions, such as anxiety, a burden of responsibility for the information and fear of a negative response. This stress can result in a reluctance to deliver the bad news. Doctors and other health-care professionals are also not immune to the experience of personal loss. A recent experience of loss or illness in our own families may make it difficult for us to break bad news to our patients and to give them support.

Whatever difficulties exist in breaking bad news to adults, they are compounded when dealing with children and young people, even though the task is often more simple and straightforward. It is worth remembering that for both parents and child, bad news might shatter hopes and dreams about the child's future.

Both the doctor and the parents eventually have to decide how to tell the child the news, and exactly what to say. If children find out unexpectedly, they can feel angry and cheated. The clinician must judge carefully how much information should be given, at which stage and by whom.

This chapter aims to provide a practical guide, incorporating the key elements of the 'breaking bad news' literature and teasing out factors that are relevant to psychiatric practice.

Literature reviews looking at patient experiences in receiving bad news suggest that there are four components that are important to this process:
1 the setting
2 the manner of the communication
3 what information is given and in how much detail
4 what support is offered afterwards.

These components vary in importance according to demographic differences, for example, younger and/or more educated patients want as much detail/

information as possible, whereas older patients may wish to know less or have their family informed instead of themselves.

We will also explore ways to facilitate breaking bad news using the framework of the Calgary–Cambridge (CC) model (Kurtz *et al.*, 2005).

SKILLS FOR YOU TO APPLY

The structure and skills of the Calgary–Cambridge (CC) model provide a secure platform for breaking bad news. For example, the approach to explanation and planning involves building supportive and trusting relationships with the patient and significant others who are present, tailoring information giving to the patient's needs, attempting to understand the patient's perspective and working in a collaborative partnership.

Finely tuned information-giving skills are most required when there is a divergence between the doctor's and the patient's perspectives. Breaking bad news is the ultimate example of such a situation. Here, the patient's hopes on entering the room are focused on the possibility, however faint, of receiving good news and the doctor has to gradually move the patient's attention towards the worrying facts that he must now begin to communicate.

This is the one communication issue that most clinicians appreciate to be a problem and find difficult. The psychological sequelae of breaking bad news in an abrupt and insensitive way can be devastating and long lasting. Over the years, there have been numerous articles in the lay and medical press that illustrate clinicians' deficiencies in this area. Nevertheless, an increasing number of publications on teaching about breaking bad news have also appeared in mainstream health education, reflecting the importance of this issue to both learners and teachers.

Clinicians may well have to tell patients that they have a serious condition, for example, bipolar affective disorder, schizophrenia or dementia. More frequently, doctors have to tell the patient news that the practitioner may not consider to be particularly important or 'bad', but which the patient or the patient's family does perceive to be so. Examples could include giving a diagnosis of attention deficit hyperactivity disorder (ADHD), or even telling a patient with an eating disorder who wishes to go on holiday the next day that they have again lost weight and are unlikely to be well enough to travel. We are often unaware of the importance of our information giving to the patient and its likely effect.

In the context of disclosing bad news, the skills of establishing a common ground, acknowledging and responding sensitively to the patient's perspective (thoughts and feelings), and demonstrating attentive verbal and non-verbal behaviour are the building blocks for creating and sustaining therapeutic relationships, regardless of whether clinician and patient are virtual strangers or know each other well.

Here the skills of the Calgary–Cambridge (CC) model will have to be applied with greater depth, intention and intensity because breaking bad news is a context that changes both the content of the interview and the intensity, intention and awareness with which certain of these core communication skills need to be applied. Below is a description of these process skills under the appropriate headings.

There are five phases in CC skills for this area:

1 **Preparing and establishing initial rapport**. Here, it is worth considering to:
   — Pay attention to seating arrangements and greetings, ensure privacy, avoid interruptions (turn off mobiles and pagers), establish the identities of everybody present and put aside your own baggage.
   — Be familiar with all aspects of the information and any diagnosis; rehearse what you might want to say and the answers to likely questions.
   — Check the patient is accompanied by someone. If not, consider whether they would like anyone with them.
   — Gauge the patient's initial comfort level with you and adjust your approach accordingly.
   — Attend to the comfort of all members of the family and establish what the patient and family already know about the problem.
   — Check for non-verbal cues to identify points at which the patient wants to ask a question:
     • Clinician: *I feel that you are very distressed to see your son staying in his room, talking to himself and behaving strangely . . .* (pause) *Have you got any concerns you wish to discuss now?*
     • A special case of picking up cues is associated with a point at which the patient (or relative/friend/significant other) who is receiving bad news seems to block out or be unable to take in what the clinician is saying. This is commonly known as shutdown. Acknowledging that the patient does not want to hear any more requires chunking and checking of information giving as the clinician proceeds, paying particular attention to the patient's non-verbal cues (such as becoming tearful, silent or looking uncomfortable).

2 Then, we should move on to **gathering information**, trying to:
   — Discover what the patient already knows (or suspects), what he/she is fearful of and he/she is hoping for.
   — Be prepared! Make sure you know about the patient's clinical condition and have read his/her records.
   — Develop an awareness of the patient's emotional state.
   — Discover what the patient wants to know. A direct preliminary question, such as *If these problems turn out to be something a bit serious, are you the type of person who likes to know exactly what is going on?* could be of assistance to accomplish this.

— An alternative approach might be to paint different scenarios, pausing after each one to gauge the patient's reaction, or using euphemisms, i.e. utilising a lighter word or phrase instead of one potentially worrying, unpleasant or hurtful, such as *Getting confused at times* instead of *He does not even know where he is.*

— Ensure that the patient feels listened to, that their information and views are welcomed and valued.

— Actively encourage a shopping list of problems in the patient's own words, using open and closed questioning techniques.

— Determine and acknowledge the different ideas present in the family, since beliefs about the cause of illness may differ, and establish all perspectives.

— Avoid jargon or technical speech and encourage the expression of feelings. Don't say *I know how you feel.* Instead, try *I think I know how you feel* or, if it is the case, *I cannot even start to imagine how it must feel for you right now.*

3 Then, we need to structure the interview by **summarising and signposting**, especially when transferring attention between different family members.

— Summarise where things have got to, checking with the patient. An example would be: *Brian, your mother has just told me about your worries and what she thinks they are. Now I want to hear from you; can you tell me what is bothering you?*

— Giving a warning shot first is a special case of explicit signposting of information that is about to be given, alerting the patient and family that all is not as they hoped. It may be useful to give a warning shot near the beginning of the interview, particularly when it is a follow-up interview.

— Expressions such as *I am sorry, but the news isn't as good as we hoped for,* accompanied by appropriate non-verbal behaviour, followed by a pause letting the likelihood of the news being difficult for the patient to sink in, before continuing the interview, tend to work well.

— To help patients and families focus their attention, the usual signposts are also important, e.g.: *There are two important things to remember, first . . . and second . . .*

4 With regard to **explaining and planning**, we ought to:

— Provide the correct amount and type of information suitable for any member of the family to understand.

— Identify the patient's specific concerns, prioritising them and breaking them down.

— Incorporate the perspectives from different family members when giving information and in decision making.

— Provide a prognosis of the problems that the patient presents with.

- Be on the patient's side, confirming your role as the patient's advocate.
- Emphasise and illustrate with examples of how quality of life will be preserved.
- Give hope tempered with realism. Clearly, this is easier for the clinician when the patient has a real hope of recovery or improvement, for example a patient recovering from post-traumatic stress disorder after a road traffic accident, or getting over a depressive episode. It is much more difficult to give hope to a patient who is depressed after receiving a diagnosis of dementia following a severe stroke. It is therefore essential for the clinician to discover the patient's own coping strategies and to find out how optimistic a person they usually are.
- Acknowledge that you may need to repeat the information or explanations as the information may not be retained, especially if there is a high level of distress.

5 Finally, when **closing the session**, it is important to make sure that the patient and the rest of the group feel heard and understand the mechanisms that the clinician has put in place to ensure safety, to summarise and check that the patient has understood, making written information available and setting up flexible follow-up meetings. This appears to be the key to conquer parental and patient satisfaction, mobilise support systems, ensure an accurate understanding and maximise engagement.

Scenario

Brian is a 17-year-old student whose performance at college has gradually deteriorated over the last few months, missing classes and raising the concerns of his peers and teachers. He has become much less sociable and spends more and more time in his room, where occasionally his parents hear him shouting out when he is alone. Brian has made superficial cuts in his forearms. There have been significant tensions within the family for the last 3 months, and Brian has withdrawn from his friends. When they have tried to contact him by telephone, he has refused to speak with them.

Brian believes that there is nothing wrong with him and is convinced that there is a conspiracy to stop him getting good grades. He states that if he is anxious and agitated, it is because his head of year is planning to stop him getting into a university course.

On interview, Brian says that he has heard the teachers commenting on his thoughts: *He is never going to make it . . . We'll give him a low mark for this essay.* Brian explains that he can hear these conversations going on outside his head and that the voices he hears are as real as the voice of the clinician interviewing him. He appears to be very fixed about these beliefs.

Brian also comes across as suspicious about his family and questions their motivations. He feels unable to go to class because he believes his peers and his teachers *have got it in for me*, and that they are always talking about him behind his back.

Brian's parents are increasingly concerned about him and say that they feel he is mentally unwell. They disclose that Brian has started to carry a knife with him, for protection, and he has become increasingly aggressive towards them. They explain that he has also become very irritable with his 11-year-old brother, giving him peculiar looks. On reflection, his parents say that Brian has been behaving oddly for the last 9 months.

HOW TO DO IT

The key tasks are:

1 Identify why it is difficult to break bad news.
2 Describe the process of giving bad news.
3 Consider what to do if the patient lacks insight.
4 Describe how to break bad news to children.
5 Can we use words that are likely to induce fear when breaking bad news?

Task 1: Identify why it is difficult to break bad news

When approaching the question *Why is it difficult to break bad news?*, the themes that keep appearing when discussing this issue with experienced clinicians or when reviewing critical incident reports are:

➤ the messenger may feel responsible and fears being blamed
➤ clinicians being unsure about the diagnosis
➤ not knowing how best to do it
➤ possible inhibition because of personal experience of loss
➤ reluctance to change the existing doctor-patient relationship
➤ fear of upsetting the patient's existing family roles/structure
➤ not knowing the patient, their resources and limitations
➤ fear of the implications for the patient, e.g. academic, social or financial losses, and of the patient's emotional reaction
➤ uncertainty as to what may happen next and worry about not having answers to some questions
➤ lack of clarity about one's own role as a health-care provider
➤ who the news is being broken to; Brian or his parents? (in our scenario), since they may have very different perspectives on what is happening, and both need attending to
➤ the patient may not think he is unwell but has an alternative explanation for what is going on; the patient may therefore be unlikely to accept your

explanation because he might struggle marrying two very different points of view.

Task 2: Describe the process of giving bad news

The process of giving bad news involves:

➤ preparing yourself
➤ giving information
➤ checking the patient's understanding of the information
➤ identifying the patient's main concerns
➤ eliciting the patient's coping strategies and personal resources
➤ giving realistic hope
➤ avoiding statements and false reassurances that have been made many times in similar situations
➤ providing support.

There are five key stages in the process of breaking bad news:

1 Before you start
   — Confirm all the information for yourself and ensure that you have all the information to hand, if necessary.
   — Speak to other professionals involved to get background information on what the patient knows, their fears, and details of the relationship with any family or friends who may be present.
   — Remember the general principles of practice: avoid jargon and speak slowly and clearly.
   — Be aware that the patient may break your prepared flow of information, requiring you to think on your feet. If asked a direct question, honesty and being straightforward is the best policy.
2 Choose the right place and ensure the right people are present
   — Pick a quiet, private room where you will not be disturbed.
   — Ensure there are no pieces of furniture between you and the patient.
   — Arrange the chairs so that everyone can be seen equally.
   — Switch off your mobile phone or leave it with someone else.
   — Invite another member of your team who knows the patient to join you.
   — Consider if the patient would like anyone present.
3 Establish the patient's previous knowledge and how much they want to know
   — Questions such as *What do you think is the matter with you?* or *What have other clinicians told you?* might help.
   — Before breaking bad news, you need to establish what the patient actually wants to hear. Open questions such as *Have you thought about what might be the cause of these problems?* or *Do you know why we referred you*

to the early intervention team? (or to the memory clinic, etc.) could also help.

— Establish how much information the patient is likely to want to know. *If this condition turns out to be something serious, are you the type of person who likes to know exactly what is going on?* It is acceptable to ask directly if they want to hear what you have to say: *Are you the sort of person who likes to know all the facts?*

— If the patient has a very different view of what is wrong, try and establish some common ground and use that to help them understand your explanation for what is happening.

4 Consider warning shots and allow time for information to sink in

— Break news in a step-wise fashion, delivering multiple warning shots. This gives the patient a chance to stop you if they have heard enough, or to ask for more information.

— Keep your sentences short, clear, and simple. A conversation may develop like this:

> Patient: *What do you mean, 'more serious'?*
> Clinician: *Well, you have been very forgetful lately . . .*
> Patient: *Do you mean that I have dementia?*
> Clinician: *Well, this is certainly a diagnosis that we need to consider.*

— At any point, the patient can stop you, signalling that they do not want to hear more about it. Less experienced clinicians sometimes feel that they must tell the patient 'the full story'. The lesson here is to respect the patient's coping strategies.

> Clinician: *I'm afraid the test results show that things are more serious than we first thought.*
> Patient: *Just tell me what we can do next.*

— Allow time for each piece of information to sink in and assume that the patient will not remember (even if the problem is not dementia) the exact details of what you have said, prompting the need to repeat important information and schedule another meeting in the not-too-distant future to continue the conversation.

— Wait in silence to let the information sink in. If emotionally distressed, the patient will not be receptive to what you say next. The moment after the bad news has been broken is uncomfortable, and you should fight the temptation to move to a more positive approach (something on the lines of *The good news is . . .*) too quickly.

End with summarising the information, check understanding and repeat any information as needed, allowing time for questions and making arrangements for follow-up.

In addition, questions such as these might be of assistance:

— *If you were upset or frightened, who would look after you and make sure that you were all right?*
— *If you do something well, who would be proud and praise you?*
— *Is there anyone else who ought to know you are here today?*
— *Is there anyone whom you would be afraid to share the news with?*
— *Has anyone in the family suffered from a similar problem?*
— *Who finds it most difficult to cope?*
— *What ideas do* (different family members) *have about* (the disorder that the patient suffers from)?
— *Whose views about health and treatments are most influential in your family?*
— *Do you understand everything that we have discussed?*
— *Is there anything that you would like to ask me?* (at the ending stage)

Task 3: Consider what to do if the patient lacks insight

In many psychiatric conditions, especially the most serious, patients when acutely unwell do not feel that they are ill but have an alternative belief as to why they are experiencing their problems. In our scenario, Brian believes that there is a conspiracy perpetrated by the college staff to stop him from getting good grades. He is, therefore, unlikely to accept the suggestion that in fact he is unwell and that whilst his experiences seem very real to him they are actually part of the illness.

We can break down what to do when the patient lacks insight into four stages:

1 **Establishing a good rapport** will be crucial at the outset and validating their experiences without necessarily agreeing with them.

Statements that might help to achieve this could be:
— *I understand that what you are experiencing is very real to you.*
— *You clearly believe what you are telling me.*
— *I can see that you are very distressed by what is going on.*

2 **Information gathering** in order to understand how they are affected by what they believe is happening to them. How do they think a doctor or health professional can help? Trying to establish something that both the clinician and the patient can work with can be useful, as it gives both parties something to agree with and start from.

For example:
— *I can see that you are very distressed at the moment and perhaps we can help with that.*
— *I wonder how you are sleeping these days.*
— *I expect you are worried about your grades.*

3 **Explanation and planning.** Once you have established some common ground, it may be possible to start introducing an alternative explanation for

the patient's experiences that they may find easier to accept. We could use expressions such as:

— *Sometimes when people are very stressed, they start to experience things happening to them that do not make sense to other people.*
— *When people are not sleeping very well, they can start hearing or seeing things that other people don't. Do you think that could be happening to you?*
— *Anxiety and lack of sleep affect everyone and can lead to unusual experiences that are difficult to explain, even looking as if someone is losing touch with reality. These experiences can seem very real. Do you feel that something like this could be behind what you feel is happening around you?*

This can then lead on to breaking the news that they are ill and agreeing on a treatment plan together.

4 **Closing the session** once this has been done by summarising the discussion, checking understanding and repeating as necessary.

In some cases, it is not possible to give a full explanation and diagnosis at this point, but it is important to have started the process and to have done so as far as possible with the patient, as this avoids disengagement later and possible further deterioration. This can be helped by providing appropriate and understandable information in frequent small doses.

Task 4: Describe how to break bad news to children and young people

The conversation with child, young person and parents should cover all basic information, consequences of the information, including likely behavioural reactions, the effects that this may have on relationships and the different members of the family's beliefs about the problems.

Such conversation could be illustrated in the following dialogue with Brian (from our scenario) if the clinician was thinking about an admission to an adolescent inpatient unit.

We will split it in four sections: basic information, behaviour in relation to the statement, effects on relationships, and beliefs and fears.

(a) Basic information:

Clinician: *I wonder if taking you away from your current situation and giving you some thinking space in a different environment might help you to unwind and look at all the stressful things that have been going on from a different angle?*

(b) Behaviour in relation to the statement:

Clinician: *Have you been to a young people's unit before?*

Brian: *No.*

Clinician: *The way it works is, I would speak and write a letter to the team who run the unit. Then, they would invite you to visit them and check them out. If you felt all right about the place and the people, they would invite you to get some things from home and go back. What would you like to bring with you if you were to come into the unit?*

(c) Effect on relationships:

Brian: *I do not want to go to the stupid unit. It's the teachers who should go there.*

Clinician: *Well, unfortunately this is not possible, but just think for a minute what could you not be without.*

Brian: *My laptop, my iPod and my mobile phone. I would also want to see my parents.*

Clinician: *Of course your parents would be able to visit. Who else would you miss?*

Brian: *Not my brother. He knows something and does not want me to go to uni, but who would feed my dog?*

Clinician: *I did not know you had a dog! What is his or her name?*

Brian: *Bolt.*

Clinician: *So when your parents visit, they could bring Bolt and you maybe could even take him for a walk if you want.*

(d) Beliefs and fears:

Brian: *Will this mess get sorted out? Will we get to the bottom of it?*

Clinician: *I hope so. First we'll try to find out what is the matter, and we will consider your thoughts about why this is happening as well.*

Brian: *My nan died in hospital.*

Clinician: *Sometimes people get very sick and can die in hospital. Are you worried about something happening to you?*

Brian: *I don't know how far they'll go . . .*

This could link back with (a) and gathering basic information around going into hospital.

Task 5: Can we use words that are likely to induce fear?

There are certain words which are likely to generate fear, such as 'psychosis', 'schizophrenia' and 'dementia'. The clinician should only use these if he is sure that the patient wants to know the full story. However, it is very important to be aware that by avoiding these words one could be causing confusion. It is clear that by using certain words people will instinctively assume that the clinician means something more serious.

Top tip

Use your **ABCDE** (used with permission of Dr Vandekieft, 2001):

*A*dvance preparation
*B*uilding relationship
*C*ommunicate well
*D*ealing with relationships
*E*ncouraging/validating emotions

OSCE practice task 13

Referring to the information included in this chapter about Brian and his parents and spending up to 10 minutes per task:

1 Explain the condition to Brian's parents.

2 Summarise how you would break bad news in mental health, covering the areas of preparation, beginning the session, sharing information, being sensitive to the patient, planning and supporting the patient, and closing the session. Please provide at least four aspects that you would consider for each of them.

3 List 10 aspects that you would take into consideration when breaking bad news to children or young people.

REFERENCES

Kurtz SM, Silverman JD, Draper J. *Teaching and Learning Communication Skills in Medicine.* 2nd ed. Oxford: Radcliffe; 2005.

Vandekieft GK. Breaking bad news. *Am Fam Physician.* 2001; **64**(12): 1975–8.

FURTHER READING

Buckman R. *How to Break Bad News: a guide for the healthcare professional.* 1st ed. London: Papermac; 1994.

Harrison ME, Walling A. What do we know about giving bad news? A review. *Clin Pediatr.* July 2010; **49**(7): 619–26.

Kraman SR, Hamm JC. Risk management: extreme honesty may be the best policy. *Ann Intern Med.* 1999; **31**: 963–7.

Mauritz M, van Meijel B. Loss and grief in patients with schizophrenia: on living in another world. *Arch of Psychiat Nurs.* 2009; **23**(3): 251–60.

McCulloch P. The patient experience of receiving bad news from health professionals. *Prof Nurse.* 2004; **19**(5): 276–80.

Ptacek JT, Eberhardt TL. Breaking bad news: a review of the literature. *JAMA.* 1996; **276**(6): 496–502.

Schmid Mast M, Kindlimann A, Langewitz W. Recipients' perspective on breaking bad news: how you put it really makes a difference. *Patient Educ Couns.* 2005; **58**(3): 244–51.

CHAPTER 11

Mental health consultations in primary care: managing the 'heartsink patient'

Jane Calne and Lisa Jackson

LEARNING OUTCOMES

- Develop advanced listening skills to pick up cues and clues in these patients
- Develop appropriately timed questioning skills to unravel the context in which the 'heartsink patient' presents their symptoms
- Develop appropriate skills in providing reassurance, explanation and planning to break the cycle of symptom presentation and investigation

INTRODUCTION

In this chapter, we have attempted to synthesise much of the advice and suggestions from the earlier chapters in the book and demonstrate how good communication skills can help in managing patients who can present major problems to health professionals. This chapter is based around consultations in primary care. In order to demonstrate clearly the communication skills employed and their effect on the patient, this section contains examples of much longer dialogues than in previous chapters. Although these communication skills are applicable to all members of the multidisciplinary team, the examples given relate to doctor-patient consultations in general practice.

WHY IS IT IMPORTANT TO UNDERSTAND COMMUNICATION SKILLS FOR DEALING WITH THE 'HEARTSINK PATIENT'?

It is important to understand how to use more advanced communication skills with the heartsink patient because it can greatly improve the satisfaction gained by both the patient and the clinician from the consultation. In the long term, this may enable the patient to manage their condition better, leading to overall improvement in their physical and psychological health. Since such patients have traditionally had a negative effect on the clinician's emotions, understanding a better way of dealing with these types of consultations may also improve the health professional's psychological health and decrease the levels of stress in their working lives.

WHO IS THE HEARTSINK PATIENT?

The term 'heartsink patient' was first used in relation to general practice by O'Dowd in 1988. The term arises from the negative emotional reaction induced in the clinician during the consultation. There have been several studies on the reasons for the negative experience that the clinician has with this particular type of patient, and various theories have been suggested as to why some primary care practitioners appear to have more of these patients than others in the same practice. Clinicians who perceive that they have more heartsink patients than others tend to be under more stress, feel that they are underperforming, have fewer postgraduate qualifications and, most importantly, have not had further training in communication or counselling skills (Mathers *et al.*, 1995).

SO WHY DOES THE CLINICIAN'S HEART SINK WHEN THESE PATIENTS' NAMES APPEAR ON THE LIST FOR THE DAY'S CONSULTATIONS?

The heartsink patient frequently consults the same health-care professional with numerous symptoms, some of which are medically explained and some which are not. They tend to cause sufficient diagnostic uncertainty to generate numerous investigations and referrals to secondary care. However, as soon as one line of enquiry is completed, another round of problems seems to present, usually as physical symptoms that are distressing and worrying to both the patient and the clinician. It often feels as if both patient and clinician are on a merry-go-round of symptom presentation and referrals with a sense that neither of them quite gets to the root of the problem. This leaves the clinician feeling impotent and the patient continuing to present with unresolved symptoms. It is estimated that an individual British GP would have about six heartsink patients, but the range is wide, between one and fifty, suggesting perception may be a factor (Butler and Evans, 1999).

During training we are taught to make diagnoses and find solutions, and when we cannot do this we can end up feeling very frustrated and unhappy. Even before one of these patients enters the room, the clinician's heart has already started to sink in anticipation of the frustration and likely unresolved outcome. The cumulative effect of many similar previous consultations with the patient induces a cycle of negative expectation for both clinician and patient.

The heartsink patient seems to engender a sense of confusion and frustration in health-care professionals in a way that other patients who are difficult to help do not. For example, a patient with chronic depression can be difficult to support, but there is a sense in the consultation that there has been a therapeutic interaction for which the patient is grateful, even though they are not better. Similarly, following the consultation, a patient with cancer will often feel better from a psychological viewpoint, even though the clinician is unable to cure the patient.

Unlike other patients, heartsink patients do not seem to get a sense of closure or ever feel properly reassured. This is clear from both their non-verbal behaviour (looking unhappy or worried, head down or shaking their head after they have been told everything is normal) and utterances such as *If only we could get to the bottom of this* or *I shouldn't have to put up with this*. There is often a hidden criticism of the clinician in these statements which may make his heart sink even further (e.g. *Why haven't YOU found out what is wrong?*). This leads to the cycle of investigations, consultations, explanations and further investigations which causes increasing dependence. This is usually focused on one particular clinician who *understands my case and everything I've been through*. These patients will wait to see this practitioner even if he is on holiday. Long-term frequent consultations like this with the same patient lead to a tremendous dissatisfaction for the clinician, when even just contemplating the consultation. The continual reliance by the patient on that staff member to solve all their problems can be very emotionally draining.

We believe that by learning to develop the skills of the Calgary–Cambridge model, it is sometimes possible to break the cycle of symptoms. Understanding the context in which the patient presents the symptoms is crucial, as it finally allows the clinician empathy with his patient. The shared understanding for both patient and clinician leads to greatly improved satisfaction in future consultations and the heartsink patient consultation can be transformed into a heartfelt understanding of what is going on for this individual.

The dividends of this are not to be underestimated for both parties. The patient becomes more self-reliant and as a result will consult less often. Reducing the number of times the clinician's heart sinks in any particular week leads to improved job satisfaction, and in the long term this in itself leads to greater well-being for the practitioner and all his patients.

SPECIAL CONSIDERATIONS FOR THIS TOPIC

1 Balancing the desire to understand context and root cause with the responsibility of not missing an important diagnosis (i.e. beware the boy who cried 'Wolf!').

2 Delicacy and sensitivity in bringing up past experiences that could be painful.
3 Time factors. In primary care, appointments usually last 10 minutes; clinicians may need to plan a longer appointment in order to address the underlying issues.
4 Patients in general practice cannot be discharged, unlike hospital practice. This makes it all the more important to attempt to change the negative heartsink response where possible.

SKILLS FOR YOU TO APPLY

1 Gathering information: especially social background, context and family history.
2 Past medical history: may be extremely relevant, patient and patient's family's experience of illness.
3 ICE: *Ideas* and *Concerns* – relating these symptoms to previous personal experiences or experiences of people close to the patient; *Expectations* regarding what the clinician can realistically do for the patient.
4 RAV: *Recognising* where the worry regarding uncertainty has come from, *Acknowledging* this, *Validating* and showing empathy.
5 Explanation: of likely cause of the intense worry regarding the symptoms and future planning for dealing with this worry.

Scenario

Sandra Bunion, a 69-year-old retired teacher, has booked into your afternoon surgery at short notice, having requested a double appointment with you. She had refused an earlier appointment with another partner. Her husband, Bill (aged 63), usually attends with Sandra, and he always brings a large plastic shopping bag with what looks like some papers and smaller bags of medication within. Sandra is well known to you: she has been attending the surgery since you joined 15 years ago and generally sees you. If you are away, she will wait until your return rather than see another partner. She has a few medical problems, including hypothyroidism diagnosed 5 years ago, intermittent vertigo, stress incontinence and mechanical back pain. She has a BMI of 31. She takes levothyroxine 100 mcg daily, 5 mg prochlorperazine PRN and co-codamol or ibuprofen. She also takes simvastatin 40 mg, cetirizine 10 mg and citalopram 20 mg daily. Her last period was 19 years ago, she had minimal symptoms around the menopause and never used hormone replacement therapy (HRT).

Bill opens the consultation. Sandra has been attending for some time with fatigue, indigestion, insomnia, generalised pruritis and intermittent paraesthesia in various parts of her body. Sandra has attended the surgery 16 times over the last 4 months, either through on-the-day or advance bookings. So far, most investigations have been normal, with only the minor elevation of thyroid-stimulating hormone (TSH 4.3; normal range 0.15–3.20 mIU/L) and thyroxine (T_4 15; normal range 8–28 pmol/l). An endoscopy carried out 2 weeks ago was normal, as was balance testing at the ENT department. Lumbar spine X-rays show minor degenerative changes, and the continence clinic has recommended pelvic floor exercises. She now presents with 'sweating at night' and a dry cough for 2 weeks.

KEY TASKS

1 Recognise and acknowledge your own feelings about the heartsink patient before they arrive in the room.

2 Once you experience your heart 'sink', see it as a challenge and prepare yourself mentally to try more advanced communication skills.

3 Ask open questions initially, e.g. *What can I do for you today?* or *How have you been?*

4 Find out how symptoms affect activities of daily living, relationships and ability to work, and how they feel about this, e.g. ask the patient to describe a typical day.

5 Ask the patient what their main concern is.

6 Ask about personal, past medical and psychological experiences and if there are any similar medical or psychological experiences in their close family or childhood, e.g. *Did you have any serious illnesses/accidents as a child? Can you tell me a bit about the family you grew up in? Were your parents and siblings healthy when you were young?*

7 Recognise the validity of their symptoms in the context of the extended picture you have gained regarding their lives.

8 Demonstrate support for their suffering.

9 Share understanding of symptoms and explain carefully what you believe to be the cause and why you do not think further tests are warranted at this time.

10 Discuss a shared plan of management and support.

Don't say:

> *There is nothing wrong with you!*
> *It's all in your head, you are depressed!*
> *I will not do any more tests, they are always negative.*
> *Do you realise how often you come to the surgery?*
> *Maybe we should arrange a total-body MRI scan?*

Try this instead:

Can you tell me about your typical day at the moment?
How do your problems affect you day to day?
Is there something that is playing on your mind about these problems?
Has any of your family had anything similar?
Was anyone in your family ill whilst you were growing up?

Dialogue example from the scenario

Bill: *Poor Sandy, she's just about had enough of all these problems, she is tired all the time, has itching, can't sleep and has indigestion and now she's had this dry cough for 2 weeks and has been sweating!*

GP: *Sandy, how do you feel?*

Sandra: *I just wish we could find out what the problem is, the cough is getting me down too now, I just don't know how to cope anymore. I don't know what I'd do without Bill.* (Turns to Bill and touches his hand and sighs, he smiles back and holds tightly onto a large carrier bag with some papers and files in.)

GP: *Is the cough getting worse?*

Sandra: *No, it's a bit better but I had some bad sweats 2 nights ago.*

GP: *I'd like to listen to your chest in a minute but first let's go through these blood tests. Fortunately they have all been very good, you are not anaemic and your kidneys and liver are working very well, your thyroid blood test was OK, we just need to monitor it to check your dose of thyroxine. What do you feel about these tests?*

Sandra: *Well to be honest I did hope that one of them would explain why I've been so tired. I just want to know what's been wrong with me, surely there are some more tests you could do?*

GP: *I am just not sure at the moment that that is the right thing to do as it seems that we have put you through a lot lately, including the telescope in your stomach and the balance test for your dizziness. I think we need to take some time here and think about what is really going to help.*

Sandra: *I heard that in America you can have a total body scan to make sure nothing is lurking, do you think that would be a good idea?* ('Lurking' is a cue.)

GP: *We can't do that here, I'm afraid, and I'm not sure it's the best thing for you. When you said you wanted to be sure that nothing was lurking, is there anything that you think it might be?* (Responds to cue re lurking but does not respond to idea of further tests, which would keep the cycle going.)

Sandra: *I don't know, you can't be sure by just examining, can you?*

GP: *Let's just look at your chest, shall we?* (Always important to do a physical examination for a new symptom and helps reassure and give reassuring 'laying on of hands' to patient.)

> GP: *Good, that's completely clear. No wheezes or extra noises that shouldn't be there.*

(Sandra still looks worried despite the reassurance from the examination. This is a non-verbal clue that she is not happy. As she is one of your heartsink patients, you are not surprised but decide to try a different approach today as you have a bit more time because the next patient has cancelled.)

> Bill: *Poor Sandra, she has suffered so much!*
> GP: (Pauses and thinks whilst watching Bill and Sandra. GP looks at Bill and notices the bag he has been carrying with files in, realises that he has had it with him the last few times but didn't notice it properly till this moment. The bag could be a clue!) *I see you have that bag again with files in, do you mind if I ask what it is?* (Responds to the clue with hesitant sensitivity.)
> Bill: (Looks a bit sheepish) *It's a file I've been keeping with Sandy's temperature and blood pressure recordings. She tells me each time she gets a new problem and I write it down. We've been doing this at home for a while just to monitor things. Sandy asked me to do it. I did show the hospital doctors last time she was seen there but they didn't seem interested so I wasn't sure if you would be.*
> GP: *Can I see them?*

(Bill passes them over and you find several years of charts and graphs showing her temperature, blood pressure and annotated with minor symptoms. You hide your amazement at what has been going on and remain professional.)

> GP: *Goodness, Sandra, these are very well kept! How does it feel to have everything monitored like this?* (Gathering more information regarding the context and meaning for the patient.)
> Sandra: *It is reassuring and I think it might make it easier for the doctors if I got really bad. I used to do it for my children when they were young.*
> GP: *Really, what made you do that?* (Following up the lead with gathering more information.)
> Sandra: *My mum used to do it for us kids. She was a nurse, you see.*
> GP: *Oh, I see. Is there anything on the charts that worries you?* (Checking the patient's concerns.)
> Sandra: *Yes, two nights ago when I was sweating a lot.*
> GP: *What does sweating mean to you?* (Checking the patient's interpretation.)
> Sandra: *Well . . .* (pauses then blurts out) *Doctors can miss pneumonia, you know!*

GP: *Oh yes, sometimes it is difficult. Have you ever had pneumonia?* (Aware that this is a very important clue by the way she blurts it out, he follows it up carefully.)

(Sandra looks upset and starts to cry. Bill comforts her.)

GP: *Do you want a minute?* (Recognises the need for time because of the overt emotion.)

Sandra: (In between sobs) *No, it's ok. It's just that my sister died of pneumonia when she was eight, she had measles you see, it was very bad, my mum never got over it.* (This revelation is the background to the context in which this heartsink patient has presented and makes all the difference to the doctor's ability to understand and empathise with her situation.)

Sandra then tells you how her mum never recovered mentally after her daughter's death and Sandra ended up doing a large part of the caring for her four other younger siblings. The doctor talks through these events with careful reflection and compassion, showing recognition, acknowledgement and validation of these experiences, even though they had happened a long time ago.

GP: *It was very helpful to talk about what happened to your sister, even though I know it was hard for you.* (Recognise, acknowledge, validate and empathise.)

It may be that your worries about your cough and the sweating have been made worse because of this memory. (By suggesting this to the patient, it helps her to link the context of this memory with the current problem. This is a new type of explanation for this patient which could give her new insight into the problem: it has definitely done so for the doctor!)

I am happy with your chest at the moment and there are no signs of pneumonia, but if you feel any worse, please get in touch. (Reassuring and safety netting.)

Sandra: *Thank you, doctor, I feel a lot better already. It helps to know that you understand about this. Do you think Bill needs to carry on with the charts?* (The patient is showing gratitude for depth of understanding. By asking about the charts, there is some suggestion of a move away from illness behaviour.)

GP: *I think it might help you both if you didn't focus too much on those recordings at the moment. What do you think?* (Giving patient permission to move away from illness behaviour but getting them to take responsibility too and be more self-reliant.)

Bill: *It does take a lot of time and somehow we haven't done the things we thought we'd have time for in our retirement.* (A move forwards to more positive well-being ideas.)

GP: *Let's see how it goes. Can you make an appointment in 2 weeks just so I can check up on you?* (A planned follow-up consultation after the dramatic revelation that will enable some encouragement towards well-being. After this appointment, the doctor may be able to further reduce the frequency of visits.)

Sandra: (Smiling, this is the first time you have seen this in years.) *Yes doctor, thank you so much for your help!*

Summary

At the end of this long consultation, the doctor has found a way to see the context in which the patient has presented, which involved some gathering of information from the past. It is not that hard as long as cues and clues are looked for and responded to in a sensitive way. As the patient leaves, the doctor has a sense of satisfaction that he has made a positive difference this time. This is the opposite of the sinking heart he had felt when she first walked in!

Top tips for this topic

1   Keep an open mind regarding diagnosis and underlying factors and their interplay. Do not rule out diagnoses just because you have found an emotional link to the worry. Clinicians have to live with some uncertainty but should always be alert for changing symptoms. Always examine the patient; it is very hard to reassure if you don't do this vital part of the consultation.

2   Ration investigations; try to make each investigation answer a question. Satisfy yourself that you have done your best to exclude serious and unusual conditions and trust your experience to guide you. It is not possible to exclude every single disease.

3   Empathy is the key to changing the feeling of heartsink to 'heartfelt understanding' of the patient. Clinicians' attitudes will change as a result of understanding the context and the personal significance of the symptoms, and as a result they will no longer feel impotent in the consultation.

4   Keep alert for cues and clues in these patients, e.g. offhand remarks, such as: *I had a friend who had a bad pain there.* Pause after these types of cues to enable the patient to elaborate. This could also allow you to follow up with a further question, for example: *Oh what was his problem?* You may get: *He died,* or *He had Crohn's disease,* etc.

5   Keep supporting the patient even if a shared understanding of context is not achieved at first. It is useful for a therapeutic relationship and offers a chance that other cues and clues may be picked up at a later date.

OSCE practice task 14

Instructions for candidate

You are an FY2 doctor in primary care. You have been asked by your trainer to see John, a 27-year-old man with abdominal pain, in order to let him know that a recent blood screen and colonoscopy were normal. Your task is to explain that further investigation is unlikely to be useful, assess John's mental state and, based on the results, suggest an alternative management plan.

You have 10 minutes for this task.

REFERENCES

Butler C, Evans M. The 'heartsink' patient revisted. *Brit J Gen Pract*. 1999; **49**: 230–3.

Mathers N, Jones N, Hannay D. Heartsink patients: a study of their general practitioners. *Brit J Gen Pract*. 1995; **45**: 293–6.

O'Dowd T. Five years of heartsink patients in general practice. *BMJ*. 1988; **297**: 528–30.

FURTHER READING

Stuart MR, Lieberman JA. *The Fifteen Minute Hour*. 2nd ed. Philadelphia, PA: Elsevier; 2002. www.gp-training.net/training/communication_skills/consultation/heartsink.htm

Calgary–Cambridge guides

Calgary–Cambridge guide one: interviewing the patient

Initiating the session

ESTABLISHING INITIAL RAPPORT

1 **Greets** patient and obtains patient's name

2 **Introduces** self, role and nature of interview; obtains consent if necessary

3 **Demonstrates respect** and interest, attends to patient's physical comfort

IDENTIFYING THE REASON(S) FOR THE CONSULTATION

4 **Identifies** the patient's problems or the issues that the patient wishes to address with appropriate **opening question** (e.g. *What problems brought you to the hospital?* or *What would you like to discuss today?*)

5 **Listens** attentively to the patient's opening statement, without interrupting or directing patient's response

6 **Confirms list and screens** for further problems (e.g. *So that's headaches and tiredness; anything else . . .?*)

7 **Negotiates agenda**, taking both patient's and physician's needs into account

Gathering information

EXPLORATION OF PATIENT'S PROBLEMS

8 **Encourages patient to tell the story** of the problem(s) from when first started to the present in own words (clarifying reason for presenting now)

9 **Uses open and closed questioning technique**, appropriately moving from open to closed

10 **Listens** attentively, allowing patient to complete statements without interruption and leaving space for patient to think before answering or go on after pausing

11 **Facilitates** patient's responses verbally and non-verbally, e.g. use of encouragement, silence, repetition, paraphrasing, interpretation

12 **Picks up** verbal and non-verbal **cues** (body language, speech, facial expression, affect); **checks out and acknowledges** as appropriate

13 **Clarifies** patient's statements that are unclear or need amplification (e.g. *Could you explain what you mean by 'light-headed'?*)

14 **Periodically summarises** to verify own understanding of what the patient has said; invites patient to correct interpretation or provide further information

15 **Uses** concise, **easily understood questions and comments**, avoids or adequately explains jargon

16 **Establishes dates and sequence** of events

ADDITIONAL SKILLS FOR UNDERSTANDING THE PATIENT'S PERSPECTIVE

17 Actively **determines and appropriately explores**:
- patient's **ideas** (i.e. beliefs re cause)
- patient's **concerns** (i.e. worries) regarding each problem
- patient's **expectations** (i.e. goals, what help the patient had expected for each problem)
- effects: how each problem **affects** the patient's life

18 **Encourages patient to express feelings**

Providing structure

MAKING ORGANISATION OVERT

19 **Summarises** at the end of a specific line of inquiry to confirm understanding before moving on to the next section

20 Progresses from one section to another using **signposting**; includes rationale for next section

ATTENDING TO FLOW

21 Structures interview in **logical sequence**

22 Attends to **timing** and keeping interview on task

Building relationship

USING APPROPRIATE NON-VERBAL BEHAVIOUR

23 **Demonstrates appropriate non-verbal behaviour**
- eye contact, facial expression
- posture, position and movement
- vocal cues, e.g. rate, volume, tone

24 If reads, writes **notes** or uses computer, does **in a manner that does not interfere with dialogue or rapport**

25 **Demonstrates** appropriate **confidence**

DEVELOPING RAPPORT

26 **Accepts** legitimacy of patient's views and feelings; is not judgemental

27 **Uses empathy** to communicate understanding and appreciation of the patient's feelings or predicament; overtly **acknowledges patient's views** and feelings

28 **Provides support**: expresses concern, understanding, willingness to help; acknowledges coping efforts and appropriate self care; offers partnership

29 **Deals sensitively** with embarrassing and disturbing topics and physical pain, including when associated with physical examination

INVOLVING THE PATIENT

30 **Shares thinking** with patient to encourage patient's involvement (e.g. *What I'm thinking now is . . .*)

31 **Explains rationale** for questions or parts of physical examination that could appear to be non-sequiturs

32 During **physical examination**, explains process, asks permission

Closing the session (preliminary explanation and planning)

33 **Gives any preliminary information** in clear well-organised manner, avoids or explains jargon

34 **Checks patient understanding** and acceptance of explanation and plans; ensures that concerns have been addressed

35 **Encourages patient to discuss** any additional points and provides opportunity to do so (e.g. *Are there any questions you'd like to ask or anything at all you'd like to discuss further?*)

36 **Summarises session** briefly

37 **Contracts** with patient re next steps for patient and physician

Calgary–Cambridge guide two: explanation and planning
Providing the correct amount and type of information
Aims:
➤ *to give comprehensive and appropriate information*
➤ *to assess each individual patient's information needs*
➤ *to neither restrict nor overload*

1 Chunks and checks: gives information in manageable chunks, checks for understanding, uses patient's response as a guide to how to proceed

2 Assesses patient's starting point: asks for patient's prior knowledge early on when giving information, discovers extent of patient's wish for information

3 Asks patients what other information would be helpful, e.g. aetiology, prognosis

4 Gives explanation at appropriate times: avoids giving advice, information or reassurance prematurely

Aiding accurate recall and understanding

Aims:

➤ *to make information easier for the patient to remember and understand*

5 Organises explanation: divides into discrete sections, develops a logical sequence

6 Uses explicit categorisation or signposting (e.g. *There are three important things that I would like to discuss. First . . . ; Now, shall we move on to . . .*)

7 Uses repetition and summarising to reinforce information

8 Uses concise, easily understood language, avoids or explains jargon

9 Uses visual methods of conveying information: diagrams, models, written information and instructions

10 Checks patient's understanding of information given (or plans made): e.g. by asking patient to restate in own words; clarifies as necessary

Achieving a shared understanding: incorporating the patient's perspective

Aims:

➤ *to provide explanations and plans that relate to the patient's perspective*

➤ *to discover the patient's thoughts and feelings about information given*

➤ *to encourage an interaction rather than one-way transmission*

11 Relates explanations to patient's perspective: to previously elicited ideas, concerns and expectations

12 Provides opportunities and encourages patient to contribute: to ask questions, seek clarification or express doubts; responds appropriately

13 Picks up and responds to verbal and non-verbal cues, e.g. patient's need to contribute information or ask questions, information overload, distress

14 Elicits patient's beliefs, reactions and feelings re information given, terms used; acknowledges and addresses where necessary

Planning: shared decision making

Aims:

➤ *to allow patients to understand the decision-making process*

➤ *to involve patients in decision making to the level they wish*

➤ *to increase patients' commitment to plans made*

15 Shares own thinking as appropriate: ideas, thought processes, dilemmas

16 Involves patient:
   – offers suggestions and choices rather than directives
   – encourages patient to contribute their own ideas, suggestions

17 Explores management options

18 Ascertains level of involvement patient wishes in making the decision at hand
19 Negotiates a mutually acceptable plan
    — signposts own position of equipoise or preference regarding available options
    — determines patient's preferences
20 Checks with patient
    — if accepts plans
    — if concerns have been addressed

Closing the session
FORWARD PLANNING
21 Contracts with patient re next steps for patient and physician
22 Safety nets, explaining possible unexpected outcomes, what to do if plan is not working, when and how to seek help

ENSURING APPROPRIATE POINT OF CLOSURE
23 Summarises session briefly and clarifies plan of care
24 Final check that patient agrees and is comfortable with plan and asks if any corrections, questions or other issues

REFERENCES
Kurtz SM, Silverman JD, Draper J. *Teaching and Learning Communication Skills in Medicine.* 2nd ed. Oxford: Radcliffe; 2005.

Silverman JD, Kurtz SM, Draper J. *Skills for Communicating with Patients.* 2nd ed. Oxford: Radcliffe; 2005.

Kurtz S, Silverman J, Benson J, *et al.* Marrying content and process in clinical method teaching: enhancing the Calgary–Cambridge guides. *Acad Med.* 2003; **78**(8): 802–9.

The psychiatric history

Psychiatric history

Please note that not all aspects of this will necessarily be covered in a single interview.

A. Identifying information

➤ Age
➤ Sex
➤ Marital status
➤ Employment status
➤ Race
➤ Referral source
➤ Any informant

B. Presenting complaint (PC)

➤ Reason for consultation: this is usually a direct quote from the patient or may be the concerns of the referrer where the patient does not see the problem

C. History of present complaint (HPC)

➤ Current symptoms: date of onset, duration and course, impact, severity
➤ Recent psychosocial stressors: stressful life events that may have contributed to the patient's current presentation
➤ Reason the patient is presenting now
➤ This section provides evidence that supports or rules out relevant diagnoses; therefore, documenting the absence of pertinent symptoms is also important
➤ Historical evidence in this section should be relevant to the current presentation

D. Past psychiatric history (PPH)

➤ Previous and current psychiatric diagnoses

➤ History of psychiatric treatments, including outpatient and inpatient treatment, medication, psychotherapy and social treatments (include dates, places and effects)

➤ History of psychotropic medication and ECT use. Did it work? Were there any side effects?

➤ History of previous suicide/deliberate self-harm attempts and potential lethality

➤ History of risk to others

➤ Detentions under the Mental Health Act

E. Past medical history (PMH)

➤ Current and/or previous medical problems

➤ Type of treatment, including previous prescription or over-the-counter medications, home remedies

F. Current medication (DH)

➤ What are they currently prescribed? (include doses and frequencies)

➤ Are they taking it? Are there any side effects? Are they happy with it?

➤ Include over-the-counter and alternative remedies

G. Family history (FH)

➤ Relatives with history of psychiatric disorders, suicide or suicide attempts, alcohol or substance abuse and neurological disorder (e.g. Huntington's chorea, epilepsy, etc.)

H. Social history (SH)

➤ Housing and cohabitees

➤ Source of income

➤ Support network

➤ Dependants

➤ Hobbies, interests, how they spend their time – currently and in the past

I. Drug and alcohol history

➤ Current substance use, including illicit drugs, alcohol and nicotine, caffeine, etc.

➤ Include age of first use, diary of a typical day for regularly used substances and mode of use (IV, etc.)

J. Forensic history (ForH)

➤ Details of any offences, with dates and consequences
➤ Any other risk issues or antisocial behaviours (e.g. check access to guns in a rural area)

K. Personal history (PH)

➤ Normal birth?
➤ Developmental history, including developmental milestones
➤ Family structure during childhood – best structured as a genogram
➤ History of childhood sexual, physical, emotional abuse or neglect
➤ Relationships with parental figures and siblings, including periods of separation
➤ School performance and list of schools attended
➤ Peer relationships: Bullying? Loner? Truancy? Sociable? Relationships with authority figures, e.g. teachers
➤ Age of school leaving, qualifications, did they reach potential? (versus siblings)
➤ Employment history
➤ Psychosexual development and history, sexual orientation
➤ Marital history/relationship history
➤ Offspring – current relationship and location

L. Premorbid personality

This information is best obtained from an informant who has known the patient well for some time before the onset of the illness. If this is not possible, ask questions like, *Would someone who has known you for a long time say you were . . .* ; *Would your friends describe you as . . .* Try to focus on one or two aspects from each personality grouping and then get more detail as type emerges, e.g.:

➤ Do you tend to be initially trusting of others or cautious?
➤ Tendency to bear grudges or forgive quickly?
➤ Jealous?
➤ Sociable or preference for own company?
➤ Confident in social setting or fearful of rejection/criticism?
➤ Likes to be centre of attention or prefers background?
➤ Impulsive or difficulty making decisions?
➤ Ability to cope with frustration, manage temper?
➤ Perfectionist or easy-going?

Mental State Examination

The Mental State Examination is an assessment of the patient at the present time. Historical information should not be included in this section.

General appearance and behaviour
➤ Grooming, level of hygiene, characteristics of clothing
➤ Unusual physical characteristics or movements
➤ Attitude: ability to interact with the interviewer (relaxed, cooperative, suspicious, guarded, overfamiliar, preoccupied, distracted, etc.)
➤ Psychomotor activity: agitation or retardation
➤ Degree of eye contact (avoidant, appropriate, intense)

Speech
Quality and quantity of speech:
➤ Pressure of speech: rapid speech, which is typical of patients with manic disorder
➤ Poverty of speech: minimal responses, such as answering just yes or no
➤ Loudness
➤ Tone and modulation
➤ Fluency

Mood
➤ Internal emotional tone of the patient (e.g. dysphoric, euphoric, angry, euthymic, anxious, tense)
➤ Ask about biological and psychological features of depression if not already covered in history (HPC) (sleep, appetite, anhedonia, libido, worthlessness, hopelessness, etc.)
➤ Suicidal/homicidal ideas (for parents of young children, ask specifically if they have thought about harming them)

Affect
➤ External range of expression, described in terms of quality, range and appropriateness
➤ Flat: absence of all or most affect
➤ Blunted or restricted: moderately reduced range of affect
➤ Labile: multiple abrupt changes in affect
➤ Inappropriate, e.g. laughing while talking about feeling depressed
➤ Full or wide range of affect – generally appropriate
➤ Thought – commonly subdivided into 'thought form' and 'thought content'

THOUGHT FORM
Record evidence of common thought disorders such as:
➤ Blocking: sudden cessation of speech, often in the middle of a statement
➤ Flight of ideas: accelerated thoughts that jump from idea to idea, typical of mania
➤ Loosening of associations: illogical shifting between unrelated topics
➤ 'Knight's move' thinking

- Tangential thought: thought that wanders from the original point
- Circumstantial thought: unnecessary digression, which eventually reaches the point
- Echolalia: echoing of words and phrases
- Neologisms: invention of new words by the patient
- Clanging: speech based on sound, such as rhyming and punning rather than logical connections
- Perseveration: repetition of phrases or words in the flow of speech

THOUGHT CONTENT
- Ideas of reference: interpreting unrelated events as having direct reference to the patient, such as believing that the television is talking specifically to them; may be delusional
- Overvalued ideas: preoccupying ideas not necessarily out of context with social norms and acted on relentlessly
- Delusions: abnormal, unshakeable beliefs, firmly held in spite of contradictory evidence and out of context with the patient's cultural norms (e.g. the lecturers were conspiring to get him out of the course)
- Persecutory delusions: false beliefs that others are trying to cause harm, or are, for example, spying with intent to cause harm
- Erotomanic delusions: false belief that a person, usually of higher status, is in love with the patient
- Grandiose delusions: false belief of an inflated sense of self-worth, power, knowledge or wealth
- Somatic delusions: false belief that the patient has a physical disorder or defect
- Obsessions: repetitive, stereotyped thoughts or images usually perceived as distressing. Compulsions: repeated stereotyped acts, not enjoyable and usually resisted
- Suicidal and homicidal ideation: requires further elaboration with comments about intent and planning (including means to carry out plan)
- Perceptual abnormalities
- Illusions: misinterpretations of reality
- Hallucinations in any of the five sensory modalities: auditory, visual, tactile, gustatory or olfactory. Try to classify (e.g. second- or third-person persecutory hallucination)
- Delusions may be the product of an attempt to rationalise the hallucinatory experience (secondary delusions)
- Derealisation: feelings of unreality involving the outer environment, so that the environment is experienced as flat, dull and unreal

➤ Depersonalisation: a subjective experience involving a change in the awareness of one's activity where the person feels that he is no longer his normal self, feeling unreal, as if one is 'outside' of the body and observing his own activities; depersonalisation is not a delusion

Cognitive evaluation (basic)
➤ Level of consciousness
➤ Orientation: person, place and date
➤ Attention and concentration: repeat five digits forwards and backwards or spell a five-letter word ('world') forwards and backwards
➤ Registration and short-term memory: ability to register and then recall three objects after 5 minutes
➤ Fund of knowledge: ability to name past five prime ministers, five large cities or historical dates
➤ Language skills: ability to name objects, comprehend verbal and written instructions and to write a sentence
➤ Visuospatial: ability to copy diagrams (e.g. interlocking pentagons) or to draw a clock face
➤ Calculations: subtraction of serial 7s, simple maths problems
➤ Abstraction: proverb interpretation and similarities

Insight
➤ How the patient understands his current problems, the implication of these problems and what if anything should be done about them

Judgement
➤ The ability to make sound decisions regarding everyday activities
➤ Judgement is best evaluated by assessing a patient's history of decision making, rather than by asking hypothetical questions

Reflection
It's always good practice to ask the patient if there is anything they would like to ask you at the end of your history and examination. Your evaluation may well have been very stressful for the patient and it helps them to feel that you are aware of their anxieties and fears if you give them freedom to express them. Remember your agenda may not be the same as theirs.

Formulation and summary
The key findings are brought together. An initial understanding of the reasons why certain items are particularly important in this patient's presentation is proposed as the basis to negotiate the next steps.

Differential diagnosis
➤ List each ICD-10 (or DSM-IV) diagnosis present and the evidence for or against each one.

Management plan
➤ This section should include all relevant treatment modalities, including pharmacological, physical, psychological and social aspects, including formal or informal hospitalisation.
➤ Include a risk assessment and risk-management plan.

General medical screening
➤ A thorough physical and neurological examination, including basic screening laboratory studies to rule out physical conditions, should be completed.

Laboratory evaluation
➤ Full blood count with differential
➤ Blood chemistry
➤ Thyroid function tests
➤ Screening test for syphilis
➤ Urinalysis with drug screen
➤ Urine pregnancy check for females of childbearing potential
➤ Blood alcohol level
➤ Serum levels of medications
➤ A more extensive workup and laboratory studies may be indicated based on clinical findings.

Adolescent psychosocial history: the HEEAADSSS + ICE protocol

Adolescent psychosocial history: the HEEAADSSS protocol (adapted, with permission, from Goldenring and Cohen, 1998, and Goldenring and Rosen, 2004) + ICE (Ideas, Concerns and Expectations)

- ➤ **H** – Home life, including relationship with parents and siblings
- ➤ **E** – Education or employment (including financial issues)
- ➤ **E** – Eating
- ➤ **A** – Activities, including sports (noting close friendships and relationships)
- ➤ **A** – Affect (particularly whether mood is responsive to situations, considering depression)
- ➤ **D** – Drug use (legal and illegal), including cigarettes and alcohol
- ➤ **S** – Sexuality (information on intimate relationships and sexual risk behaviours)
- ➤ **S** – Suicide, self-harm and safety (risk to others as well as risk to self)
- ➤ **S** – Sleep

+

- ➤ **I** – Ideas (on what the problems are)
- ➤ **C** – Concerns (on what the problems might entail)
- ➤ **E** – Expectations (on the consultation, the problems and the management plan)

Family tree (pedigree diagram for Kevin's family history)

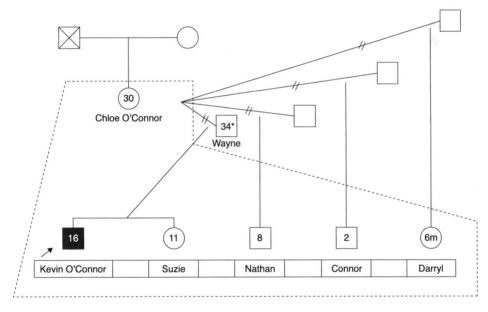

KEY

■	Affected	↗	Proband
34*	He 'drank too much' and 'got into trouble for fighting'	⫽	Indicates broken relationship
⊠	Male deceased	-------	Dashed line indicates members of household

How to pass communication skills OSCEs in mental health

The following guidance is based upon the editors' combined experience in designing and writing OSCE stations, teaching communication skills and examining both medical students and junior doctors on communication skills OSCE stations. Whilst we are focusing on communication skills in mental health settings, many of the points made here can be applied to communication skills assessments in other settings and specialties, including primary care.

Quite a lot of the information below could be summarised under the headings of 'good examination technique' and 'common sense'. Unfortunately, it is our experience that under the stress of exam conditions, common sense often 'goes out the window' and candidates sometimes do the strangest things! We hope that the following suggestions (which we have divided into 'Dos' and 'Don'ts') will help to keep you on track and prevent you stumbling into some of the commonly seen pitfalls.

DON'T:
➤ **Take too long introducing yourself.**
➤ **Assume that you can address everyone by their first name.** Check! It is always safer (particularly with older patients) to err on the side of formality. One of the older actors we use, when role-playing a retired accountant with early dementia, takes great pleasure in saying to students who address him as 'Jonathan' that *My employees used to call me Mr Brown . . .*
➤ **Promise that you will share the information with no one when discussing confidentiality** – all of the clinical team will need information and clearly there needs to be feedback to the referrer.
➤ **Appear unprofessional!** Being insensitive, rude, offhand, dismissive, condescending, unkempt, inappropriately dressed, etc. will inevitably attract poor marks. Don't forget that in some stations the actor (role-playing the patient or relative) also gives some marks for their impression of the candidate.

➤ **Undertake unnecessary tasks.** If the instructions clearly state that you do *not* need to do something, don't do it! A surprising number of candidates will, for example, start to ask the patient lots of questions about their mood when the instructions clearly state 'Mr Brown has moderate depression and wishes to discuss the different forms of treatment that are available. You do not need to take a history from the patient'. You are just sacrificing time that could be spent on gaining marks and also potentially run the risk of irritating the examiner!

➤ **Use jargon.** For example, if you are asked to explain drug treatments for depression to a patient, don't say something like *The antidepressant I would recommend for you is one of the SSRIs which work by inhibiting the reuptake of serotonin from the synapse* . . . If you have to utilise technical terms, explain them clearly in plain English. Don't forget that jargon doesn't just include scientific terms; patients often find 'NHS jargon' totally incomprehensible. For example, explaining to the relative of a patient with severe mental illness that *Because your son was admitted under Section 3 of the Mental Health Act, he will receive follow-up under the auspices of section 117 and so he will make no financial contribution towards his community care package* will mean nothing to most people.

➤ **Fire questions like a machine gun!** Although OSCEs are done under time pressure, remember that you are conducting an interview, not an interrogation. Don't ask multiple questions at the same time and allow the role player sufficient time to answer. If you need to move on or change to a different topic, signpost this clearly. For example, if the patient is getting bogged down in irrelevant details about something, you could say something like; *Mr Smith, perhaps we could come back to that in a few minutes? I would really like to ask you now about how you have been over the past week.*

➤ **Feel that you have to use all of the Calgary–Cambridge skills irrespective of the scenario.** For example, asking the patient to summarise and repeat back what you have said would be very appropriate in a station in which you were asked to provide information to a patient about to start on lithium. The same technique would probably not be appropriate in a station involving a distressed patient or an angry relative.

➤ **Collude with the patient, lie to the patient or try to 'shift the blame' onto a colleague.** Unprofessional behaviour will inevitably result in very poor marks.

➤ **Make unrealistic promises which you will be unable to keep; also, don't make promises on behalf of other health professionals.** For example, whilst you could quite properly say to a patient that you will be referring them to the Community Mental Health Team and will be asking if they can be seen quickly, you cannot promise that a community mental health nurse will visit at 9 a.m. tomorrow (unless, of course, you have already arranged this with the nurse).

➤ **Rise to provocation.** This can be an issue in scenarios dealing with angry patients/relatives or stations with psychotic or belligerent patients. Losing your temper, becoming visibly irritated or 'getting your own back' by making sharp or 'clever' comments will only wind the situation up and result in poor marks for unprofessional behaviour.

➤ **Allow the patient to take over and control (or disrupt) the interview.** This may be a particular problem with stations involving manic or disinhibited patients. Setting a clear agenda right from the start, using lots of signposting and calmly, but firmly, putting the interview back on course is the best way to proceed. This can be one of the hardest things to do in psychiatric consultations; in difficult situations you are 'walking a tightrope' between losing control of the interview on the one hand and irritating and alienating the patient by being too controlling on the other.

➤ **Give in to pressure in circumstances where you need to 'stick to your guns'.** For example, if the scenario involves an inpatient who you have assessed as having a significant risk of suicide, don't allow the patient (or a relative, if one is present in the station) to persuade you to let him leave the ward. Similarly, if the patient is clearly unwell, but is trying to negotiate a reduction in medication, remain circumspect.

➤ **Assume that all OSCE stations should have a 'good outcome' and that the patient/relative will ride off happily into the sunset.** In a station involving an angry relative or a disturbed patient, the best outcome that can be achieved may be that the situation is 'contained' (rather than escalated). Similarly, in a station with a very ill psychotic patient, it may be impossible to negotiate a mutually acceptable treatment plan. The required outcome of the station could be that you inform the examiner that an assessment under the Mental Health Act is necessary.

➤ **Panic!** If you follow the Calgary–Cambridge model and make use of the knowledge and experience you have gained throughout your training, you will do well. Hopefully this book will be of some assistance as well!

DO:
➤ **Dress appropriately** (whilst taking account of any local hospital requirements regarding ties, jewellery, being bare below the elbow, etc.). Check what happens when you bend forward (especially neck and hemline): you don't want to reveal too much about yourself – you are a health *professional*!

➤ **Arrive at least 20 minutes before the start of the OSCE.**

➤ **Behave appropriately.** Be polite, courteous and well mannered.

➤ **Read all the information and instructions relating to the OSCE station and make sure that you understand the task *before* you start.** If your mind goes blank during the station and you need to remind yourself of the scenario details or task, you will usually be allowed to review the 'information for candidates' (although this will depend upon the local rules for the examination). However, this does interrupt the flow of the station, looks less professional and costs you time.

➤ **Introduce yourself by name:** *My name is James Keen. I am a* (the role given to you in the instructions of that station). Also, ask the patient's name, if not given in the instructions.

➤ **Explain your task to the patient.**

➤ **Keep to the timing for the station: ensure you know how long the station lasts and keep a (covert) eye on the clock.** We have all seen students who have attempted to rush through a station at the speed of light because what they thought was a 5-minute station was actually allocated 10 minutes! However, there have undoubtedly been even more candidates who have just run out of time . . .

➤ **Be aware of any 'hints' from the examiner.** For example, if the examiner suggests you look at something again, do so carefully – you may be on the wrong track.

➤ **Let the examiner know you have finished.**

➤ **Remember that, if you are instructed to discuss your findings with the examiner in the last minute, you have correspondingly less time to talk with the patient.**

➤ **Call the patient/relative (or whoever you have been asked to speak with) by the correct name!** If the station instructions say 'Your task is to speak to Mr Smith . . .' and you start off by saying *Good morning, Mr Jones*, you look less capable and you also run the risk of being thrown out of your stride when the patient immediately corrects your mistake!

➤ **Ensure that you include all the actors/role players in the station.** If the instructions say that your task is 'to speak to Mr Wilson and his nurse', then make sure that you do so! Unfortunately, we have seen candidates at such stations who have completely ignored the nurse and focused on the patient (or vice versa). As a result, they failed to obtain all the necessary information about the case and were also severely marked down on their ability to undertake a triadic consultation!

➤ **Use verbal and non-verbal encouragements, such as head nods, and maintain appropriate eye contact.**

➤ **Adopt an open posture.** Sit with both feet resting on the floor. Lean forward if the situation demands it, but do not invade the patient's personal space.

➤ **Give pauses and allow the patient to talk freely for the first 30 seconds or so.**

➤ **Remember that there are marks for both process (communication skills ability/technique) and content (obtaining the desired information or explaining the required facts to the patient).** Do review the sample mark sheets in Appendix 6 as this will give you good insight into how the examiners mark these kinds of OSCE stations. You need to get a good mark for both parts. There have been candidates who have done a wonderful job of introducing themselves, made sure the patient is comfortable, reassured the patient about confidentiality, etc., but have not actually taken any relevant history whatsoever from the patient by the time the bell rang!

➤ **Follow the instructions!** If you are directed to 'discuss the pharmacological treatments available for depression' with the patient; then do just that! If you spend half the allotted time discussing CBT and only mention one antidepressant, you will not get many marks.

➤ **Adjust the volume and rate of your speech and the pace of the interview to the individual patient.** For example, to successfully interview a very depressed patient you will need to speak slowly and calmly and allow the patient plenty of time to respond. Bounding into the station with a broad smile, thrusting out your hand and saying *Hi, I'm George, one of the doctors. And how are you today?* will probably be met by a blank stare and an uncomfortable silence!

➤ **Start the consultation in an organised and controlled way.** Candidates who score good marks always start well; introducing themselves, clarifying who is present and what their expectations are and then negotiating the agenda for the consultation (including signposting how long it will last) in the first 30–60 seconds. In contrast, students who score badly almost inevitably start off in a very disorganised fashion. As a result, they never take control of the interview and it often proceeds in a very haphazard way; vital parts of the process are missed, things go off at a tangent and the consultation ends up in uncharted waters.

➤ **Show an interest in what is being said to you!** Sometimes candidates appear to be so totally preoccupied with working out what to ask next that they pay little attention to the actor and look bored or uninterested!

➤ **Try to clarify things that the patient has said that are unclear or that you do not follow.** This is particularly important with patients who may be psychotic. Asking the patient to provide an example (*What exactly did the voices say about you?*) can be extremely helpful.

➤ **Demonstrate appropriate empathy.** However, be sincere (remember that this involves using an appropriate tone of voice and body language as well as appropriate words). Patients (and actors) are very good at picking up insincerity!

➤ **Give the appearance of being familiar with the subject matter!** For example, if part of the task is to assess a patient's cognitive function, then the examiner should be able to see that you know what you are doing and have done it before. We have seen many candidates who give the appearance of never having actually undertaken a cognitive assessment and stumble through the process, asking the patient to remember a name and address but then not going back to check the patient's recall of it later on!

➤ **Prepare!** Give some thought to possible OSCE scenarios and develop a mental list of possible questions. There are certain situations, tasks and disorders in mental health that lend themselves particularly well to communication skills OSCE stations. These can be broadly divided into:

— **Information gathering** (e.g. taking a history and performing a risk assessment on a patient who has self-harmed, assessing a patient's mood state, eliciting features of psychosis from a patient, taking an alcohol/substance use history, etc.)

— **Explanation and planning** (e.g. explaining a particular diagnosis to a patient and/or relative, providing information about specific treatments for mental health conditions such as lithium and antipsychotics, etc.)

— **Complex tasks involving information gathering, information giving, negotiation and clinical judgement** (e.g. assessing mental capacity to self-discharge from hospital). These tasks will flow much more smoothly if you have spent time beforehand familiarising yourself with the different psychiatric disorders and common treatments and know what kind of questions to ask and areas to discuss. For example, if you are asked to assess someone's mood, you should immediately realise that you will also have to enquire about areas such as: sleep pattern, diurnal changes, appetite, weight, energy levels, activity patterns, the ability to take an interest and gain pleasure from life, views regarding the future, hopelessness, suicidal ideas and plans, etc.).

➤ **Think about the style of questioning**; use open questions to start: *Can you tell me what has been happening recently?* Move on to closed questions to clarify: *Whose voice was it?*; *Where did it come from?* Avoid leading questions: *So the voice you heard, was that of your neighbour coming from inside your head?*

➤ **Be safe!** If you don't know the answer or are unsure of what to do, it is better to be honest and say so. For example, it is safe to say that you would have to check a drug dose or potential drug interaction in the British National Formulary or with a pharmacist. It is dangerous to guess! Similarly, if you are unsure about whether or not a patient has the capacity to self-discharge, it is safe to say that you would keep them on the ward whilst you obtained senior guidance. Letting the patient leave if you were unsure would be dangerous! Obviously you would get a much better mark if you were able to discuss the Functional Test of Capacity and the appropriate use of the Mental Health Act and Mental Capacity Act with the examiner at the end of the station!

➤ **End by thanking the patient.** Never leave the station abruptly.
➤ **Use a rest station to calm yourself down and to think about the next station.**
➤ **Remain positive and confident.**

Example of OSCE mark sheets in mental health

STATION 1 – CONSULTATION SKILLS; INFORMATION GATHERING AND DIFFERENTIAL DIAGNOSIS; ANXIETY

Please affix candidate sticker here

MARKSHEET A: Process	Marks	Score
Introduction		
Introduces self (first and second names) and role clearly. Explains reason for interview. (No marks if rushed or mumbled.)	2	
Rapport		
Picks up cues, e.g. notices and acknowledges if patient looks or sounds worried or anxious. Expresses concern and support.	2	
Skills in eliciting information		
Listens attentively, allowing patient to use own words	2	
Uses open and closed questions appropriately	2	
Periodically summarises to check own understanding and invites patient to correct any errors	2	
Progresses from one section to another using signposting	2	
Uses clear, easily understood language, avoids jargon	1	
Structures interview in a logical sequence, attends to timing, keeps on task	2	
Involves patient in the process		
Encourages patient to express ideas, concerns, expectations, feelings and the effects on his life; responds to and further explores his perspective; shows empathy	2	
Verbally acknowledges patient's views and feelings and demonstrates appropriate non-verbal behaviour (e.g. eye contact, posture, position, movement)	2	
Provides support, expresses concern, understanding, willingness to help	2	
Actor's perspective		
The student explored my problems thoroughly	2	
The student addressed my concerns appropriately	2	
Total	**25**	

Assessor's name (please print)

Assessor's signature

Date

Overall impression

Pass

Borderline Pass

Borderline Fail

Fail

STATION 1 – CONSULTATION SKILLS; INFORMATION GATHERING AND DIFFERENTIAL DIAGNOSIS; ANXIETY

Please affix candidate sticker here

MARKSHEET B: Content	Marks	Score
Symptoms of anxiety		
Psychological / cognitive symptoms: Feelings of generalised anxiety / worry; Concerns regarding physical health / fear of serious illness / death; Feelings of impending doom; Poor concentration	4	
Physical symptoms: Sweating; Palpitations / increased heart rate; Muscular tension / tension headaches; Breathlessness / feeling unable to breathe; Feeling faint / 'dizzy' / lightheaded; Urinary frequency	6	
Behavioural changes: Agitation / restlessness; Avoidance of particular anxiety-provoking situations; Changes in social behaviour (avoiding friends); Increased alcohol use	4	
Development of illness, identifying precipitating factors and comorbidity		
Elicits when symptoms began and how they have developed over time	1	
Identifies any stressors at the time of onset	1	
Asks patient to rate severity of current problems (e.g. on a 10 point scale)	1	
Checks for any changes in mood and excludes: Feelings of depression / low mood; Sleep disturbance / changes to sleep pattern, Changes in appetite and weight; Feelings of hopelessness / worthlessness / guilt; Thoughts of suicide / self-harm	5	
Checks for history of any physical health problems	1	
Gets an idea of pre-morbid personality and normal behaviour and functioning	1	
Family history of mental health problems	1	
Diagnostic formulation / differential diagnosis presented to examiner		
Diagnosis is generalised anxiety disorder	1	
Does not fulfil diagnostic criteria for depressive illness	1	
Possible genetic / familial predisposition (strong FH of anxiety disorders)	1	
Precipitated by recent life event (death of father from heart attack)	1	
Increased alcohol use ('self medication') probably exacerbating symptoms	1	
Total	**30**	

Assessor's name (please print)
Assessor's signature
Date

Overall impression

Pass

Borderline Pass

Borderline Fail

Fail

OSCEs model answers

OSCE model answer 1

➤ Acknowledge any current symptoms the patient may be experiencing, giving them the opportunity to discuss their ideas, concerns and expectations.

➤ Ensure that, through questioning, you gain an understanding of how the symptoms started, any triggers and how the problems have developed over time.

➤ Explore with the patient the cognitive symptoms (thoughts), physical symptoms and associated behaviours. Clarify the circumstances when these symptoms occur and any environmental factors relevant in the experiencing of symptoms.

➤ Use simple rating scales, e.g. asking for a score out of 100 to understand together with the patient how severe their symptoms are now and make associations together between the severity of anxiety symptoms, physical symptoms, behaviours and functioning.

➤ Check for the presence of depressive symptoms and don't forget to assess risk of suicide or self-harm.

OSCE model answer 2

➤ Develop initial rapport, giving patients the time to express their concerns, including more specifically about how they are feeling in themselves.

➤ Explore in your questioning the patient's thoughts about their current situation, the future and past (including thoughts of guilt or regret).

➤ Link the patient's thoughts about the future to questions regarding the patient's feelings about life not being worth living and suicidal ideation and plans. It is also important to assess whether they have thoughts to harm others close to them, for example, children (particularly in post-natal depression) or partners. This clearly needs to be asked in a sensitive way.

➤ To include focused questions regarding biological symptoms of depression (sleep, appetite, weight, bowel function, libido, diurnal variation in mood).

The following may also help you to achieve your tasks:

➤ Match the pace of the interview (including verbal and non-verbal communication) to the patient.

➤ Pick up on cues to enable signposting to specific questions related to symptoms of depression and anxiety and required further questions in the Mental State Examination.

➤ Show sensitivity when the patient is disclosing difficult information with the use of appropriate empathic statements.

➤ Use of summarising, chunking and checking, repetition and paraphrasing to clarify understanding of the patient's symptoms.

➤ Being non-judgemental and supportive, both verbally (in the use of validating statements) and in the non-verbal manner of the interviewer.

OSCE model answer 3

Start with introductions, confidentiality explanation and setting the tasks for the consultation. Then explore the patient's *ideas, concerns, expectations*. For example:

Tell me what happened? Was it what you were expecting? Why did you use those tablets/that bottle? What did you think would happen?

Then summarise the patient's account of the event.

When did you first think of taking the tablets/cutting your wrist? How often have you thought about it? Had you made any preparations before you hurt yourself? Explore whether affairs put in order, note left, any other plans. Check their understanding is in line with the patient's.

How do you see the future? Do you have any other plans? Explore what the patient will do after they go home. Consider the overall picture.

Finally, summarise the information given and assess whether the patient is likely to repeat the act.

OSCE model answer 4

Remember that you only have 9 minutes for this task (as in the last minute you have to discuss the case with the assessor).

➤ Introduce yourself and explain why you are seeing the patient (e.g. *I have been told that things have become very difficult with your neighbours and that this is making you feel very stressed*).

➤ Set an agenda and signpost the interview (e.g. *Perhaps we could see if there is something that can be done to improve things? I wonder if it would be helpful to talk a bit about how things have been with the neighbours? I would like to hear your story in more detail. Then we can discuss how we can work together and make you feel a bit better. Does that sound OK to you?*).

➤ Ask the patient to describe how the difficulties with the neighbours began and how the problem has developed. Try to structure the story in chronological order if possible. Initially allow the patient to use his own words, but make a mental note of any parts of his story that will require clarification later on.

➤ If the patient is reluctant to talk, or does not know how to start, begin by asking him about how the problems he is having from the neighbours are affecting his life. You can subsequently enquire about the symptoms/experiences that he has.

➤ If the patient becomes agitated or distressed, acknowledge this and ask if they are able to continue to discuss the matter or if you should leave it for now and move onto another topic.

➤ Try to clarify as far as possible, in a sensitive manner, exactly what symptoms the patient is describing (e.g. *So, you have just told me that the neighbours know what you are thinking. Could you say a bit more about that? Perhaps you could give me an example? How does this happen exactly?*).

➤ Show appropriate empathy with the patient's difficulties and problems, but do not allow yourself to be drawn into colluding with the patient (for example, they might ask you to convince the police or the housing department that the patient is being persecuted).

➤ Given that the suggestion in the OSCE instructions is that the patient probably has a psychotic illness, go on to ask about other common features of psychosis not immediately revealed by the patient in his history (e.g. *Sometimes people have other unpleasant or strange experiences, such as hearing people talking when there is nobody else around. Have you had any experiences like that?*).

➤ Take note of any features you have observed about the patient that relate to his mental state (e.g. features of his appearance, behaviour, speech, etc.). The examiner may ask you about this at the end.

➤ If appropriate, gently assess degree of insight (e.g. *Do you think there could be any other explanation for the clicking noises you can hear on the telephone?*).

➤ The instructions specifically state that you do not have to discuss management with the patient, so do not do so! This will waste time and you will not gain marks for it.

➤ The assessor will have particular questions to ask, such as *Describe the psychotic features you have elicited.* Make sure that you do this clearly and succinctly, giving the reasons why you believe he has third-person auditory hallucinations, thought broadcast or whatever he has described.

OSCE model answer 5

You will have 9 minutes for the task.

➤ Start with an introduction explaining the purpose of the consultation

➤ Explain confidentiality with information sharing with key members of the team.

➤ Recap the symptoms described (scenario in Chapter 6):
  — Psychological testing (delusion)
  — Coded messages from the TV and newspapers (hallucinations)
  — Monitored by TV (passivity)
  — Lecturers talking about him via telepathy (thought interference)
  — Running commentary (auditory hallucination)

➤ For each, ask for his understanding of it, for example:
  — *Why do you feel they are testing you?*
  — *Have you any thoughts as to why?*

➤ Empathise with the patient and suggest the clinician's preferred management plan:
  — *Clearly it is very distressing...*
  — *Is there anything that might make it better?* Listens to the patient. Gently suggests medication.

➤ The patient is willing to accept medication.

➤ It would be usual practice to prescribe a low dose of a tablet called risperidone.

➤ *It is an antipsychotic. It will act by lowering your level of distress and reducing the interruptions from your lecturers. Some of the things that you are experiencing may be because you are unwell and the risperidone will help this. The medication works by blocking the dopamine receptors. Dopamine is one of the transmitter chemicals in the brain. Like with all medication, there are some side effects. The common ones are headaches, lowering of blood pressure and some agitation. Patients also can get constipation, feel sick, feel tired and gain weight. Less commonly, people can get blurred vision or skin rashes. Some of the side effects will wear off within a few days or weeks. Taking medication is a balance between benefits and risks.*

➤ Explain that illness requires specialist input to ensure best treatment is offered. Suggest it is important that the patient is fully assessed to treat symptoms as fully as possible: *From our discussions, you clearly realise that there has been a change and it would be best for it to be fully explored at this stage.*

➤ *Have you noticed any change in how your son is presenting?* (Allow parent the time to voice the changes and their concerns.) *Has it occurred to you that these changes might mean your son has a mental illness?* (Parent either agrees or disagrees.) Acknowledge the shock and implications of this. Time will be needed. *The Mental Health Act is there to provide care and treatment for those with an illness where the patient is not willing or is not able to see the need for treatment. I think that this is needed here to allow for a full assessment to take place in hospital as the least restrictive option.* Explain the process – need another doctor and an approved mental health practitioner: *The others will make their assessment. The AMHP has to speak with the next of kin. The Mental Health Act allows protection and rights to the patient to prevent harm.*

OSCE model answer 6

The following questions might help to explore the issues of who Kevin considers as family:

➤ *Who else knows that you are here today?*
➤ *Is there anyone else who ought to know you are here today?*
➤ *Who do you call family? / Who do you regard as your family?*
➤ *Who lives with you at home? How long have they lived there?*
➤ *Do you have your own room?*
➤ *To whom are you closest at home?*
➤ *Kevin, who cares for you and takes responsibility for you?*
➤ *Who is the most worried about you? How do you know?*
➤ *Have you tried to keep in touch with your father? What happened?*
➤ *If you were upset or frightened, who would look after you and make sure that you were all right?*
➤ *If you do something well, who would be proud and praise you?*
➤ *How many times have you moved home in the last year or so?*
➤ *What is the best thing about living where you do?* and *What is the worst thing about living where you do?*
➤ *How do you think your mother sees you managing?*
➤ *Imagine someone treated you unfairly, what would you do?*
➤ *Think of a really good time you enjoyed with your family. What was it, and what made it so special for you?*
➤ *Other than your family, who is important to you in your life?*
➤ *At home, who is working and what do they do?*
➤ *Is there enough money, from work and benefits, to meet your family's needs?*
➤ *Has anyone in the family suffered from a similar problem?*
➤ *Kevin, what does your mum think is the matter with you?* or *Chloe, what brought you to see your GP about Kevin?*
➤ *Kevin, when someone is ill at home, whose views about health and treatments are most influential in your family?*

OSCE model answer 7

The following questions might help to take a psychological history.

When considering school and educational aspects:

➤ *Kevin, what school or college do you go to? How regularly do you attend?*

➤ *What are your favourite/least favourite subjects in school?*

➤ *What might stop you going to school/college?*

➤ *What do you want to do long term? or What do you hope that learning will help you do?*

➤ *Tell me about your friends at school.*

➤ *Have you ever been suspended/expelled from school?*

To explore the activities interesting the young person:

➤ *Kevin, what do you enjoy doing with your family?*

➤ *What do you do for fun?*

➤ *What kind of hobbies (or activities) do you like doing best?*

➤ *When your mum is unwell, do you have to help to look after her or one of your brothers or sister?*

➤ *Are your friends mostly the same age as you, or are they mostly younger or older than you?*

➤ *How do you know that the people that you meet in the Internet chat rooms are who they say they are? Does it bother you? Do you meet them in real life sometimes?*

When enquiring about drug use:

➤ *Does anyone in your family smoke?*

➤ *Do any of your friends use drugs or alcohol?* (This might take the focus away from the young person.)

➤ *What kind of drugs have you seen around in your school or at parties?* (Instead of *Do you do drugs?*)

➤ *Are you aware if drugs are bought and sold in your neighbourhood?*

➤ *Do you ever drink alcohol or use drugs when you are alone?*

➤ *Do you ever use alcohol or drugs to relax?*

➤ *Do you forget things you did while using drugs or alcohol?*

➤ *Do your family and friends ever tell you that you should cut down on your drinking or drug use?*

To find out about sexuality:

➤ *You said you have been going out with _____ for the last 3 months. Has your relationship become sexual?*

➤ *Are you interested in boys/girls?*

➤ *Are your sexual experiences enjoyable?*

➤ *Have you ever been pressured or forced into doing something of a sexual nature that you did not want to do?*
➤ *Have you ever been touched sexually in a way that you did not want?*

When asking about suicide, self-harm, and issues of safety:
➤ *When you are frustrated, angry or upset, how would people around you know that something was wrong?*
➤ *Have you ever thought about hurting yourself or someone else?*
➤ *Have you ever had to hurt yourself (cutting yourself, for example) to calm down or feel better?*
➤ *Have you ever tried to kill yourself?*
➤ *Violent behaviour seems to have become more frequent for many young people. Have you ever felt unsafe at home, at school, in your neighbourhood, in a relationship, or on a date?*
➤ *Is any violence going on at home or at school?*
➤ *Have you got into physical fights in school or in your neighbourhood?*
➤ *Have you ever felt that you had to carry a knife or any other weapon to protect yourself?*

OSCE model answer 8

Kevin's family tree can be found in Appendix 4.

OSCE model answer 9

The following would be possible deadlocks when speaking with Kevin and Chloe:
➤ Chloe believes it is all down to Kevin's behaviour and that he always acts to get a reaction from people.
➤ Chloe normalises self-harm.
➤ Chloe believes that thoughts of harming others are Kevin's way to attract attention and manipulate others.
➤ Kevin does not think he has a problem.
➤ Kevin resents that his mother has always been busy with his siblings or absent as a result of her own problems.
➤ Kevin and his mother have different goals for attending the consultation.

OSCE model answer 10

The following are potential secrets that could exist in Kevin's family:
➤ parenthood of the different children
➤ Kevin's violent fantasies
➤ Kevin's use of pornographic material involving minors
➤ potential child protection concerns

➤ Kevin's resentment towards his mother, based on the belief that she has always been busy with his siblings, leaving him aside
➤ drug use
➤ issues around sexuality
➤ Kevin being seen by his mother Chloe as becoming similar to his father Wayne, who was violent towards Chloe.

OSCE model answer 11

Remember that you only have 9 minutes for this task (as in the last minute you have to discuss the case with the assessor).

➤ Introduce yourself and explain why you are seeing the patient and her daughter (*To decide how best to help you once you leave hospital* is less threatening than *To decide if you can go back home*).
➤ Set an agenda and signpost the interview (how long it will last, that you are going to address questions to the patient and to her daughter).
➤ Ask the patient how she was managing at home before hospital admission and ascertain whether she was getting any help at that time (clarify with daughter).
➤ Ask the patient and her daughter if they have noticed any changes since the fall (*Do you feel muddled/Are you having problems with your memory?*).
➤ Explain to the patient that you want to test her memory and then undertake a brief cognitive assessment using the pro forma supplied.
➤ Explore with the patient:
  — How does she think she would cope at home now?
  — Does she envisage any problems?
  — Does she think she will need any help?
  — Does she recall the OT home visit?
  — Does she agree with the OT's recommendations? (You will probably have to remind her what these were.)
  — Will she accept the help which will then allow her to return home safely?
➤ Involve the daughter in the above process. She can help to prompt and remind the patient about some issues and clarify points of fact. What is her opinion about her mother's willingness to accept help?

Discussion with examiner

➤ State whether or not you believe the patient has cognitive impairment and give your reasons (you may also say that you suspect that she has dementia, but you cannot make a definitive diagnosis on the basis of such a brief assessment).
➤ State whether or not you feel she has the capacity to make the decision to return home and explain your reasons (go through the steps from the 'functional test' of capacity).

OSCE model answer 12

1   You *are* late, so apologise. Try not to make excuses and allow Mr Beck to express his anger. For example, *I'm so sorry to be late. You must have wondered whether I was coming at all.*

2   Create an atmosphere that allows Mr Beck to feel safe enough to express his anger. Body language is crucial to show that you feel and hear both his anger and distress and that he (now) has your total attention. Look calm despite being verbally attacked and give him space to ventilate his feelings.

3   He is likely to become more enraged if he thinks you are not hearing his anger (and distress): e.g. not looking as if you are taking him seriously, or looking as if you are thinking of something else. Suggesting that you were late because you were seeing someone else (more important than Mr Beck) might be particularly inflammatory.

4   Mr Beck was adopted, so is probably sensitive to abandonment that contributed to his anxiety and depression when his girlfriend left. He is also likely to have issues with regard to developing trusting relationships. He had just begun to trust you (having revealed his adoption at your last meeting) so your being late might have felt wounding.

5   Trust your instincts: remain alert for any cues that might precede violence. Ensure that the environment is safe enough. Retain a calm demeanour to help Mr Beck feel safe. Try to remember that his anger is secondary to feeling hurt.

OSCE model answer 13

1   To explain the condition to Brian's parents, you need to consider the following:
    — Establish rapport – introduce yourself and explain why you are there.
    — Information gathering – establish what their understanding of Brian's condition is and what their worries are. (*I understand you are worried about Brian. Could you just tell me a little bit more about that? What are you worried might be wrong with Brian? Have you any ideas as to what might be going on?*)
    — Explanation – having understood what the patient's and his family's current level of understanding is, we could use this as a starting point for your explanation. (*I agree that Brian seems to be unwell and may be having a psychotic episode.*) Then take time to explain what you mean by psychosis and any treatment plan. Allow time for the parents to take in this information and gauge their reaction. Try to avoid using jargon and words that may induce fear without avoiding the truth. Leave time for them to ask questions and clarify details as necessary.
    — Planning – outline any treatment that Brian needs and the likely prognosis of Brian's difficulties.

— Close the session by summarising the discussion and plan, checking with Brian's parents that they have understood, allowing time for additional questions. Check with them that you have covered everything they wanted to know.

2 Summary of suggestions for breaking bad news in mental health:
   — Preparation
      • Set up an appointment as soon as possible.
      • Allow enough time and ensure no interruptions.
      • Use a comfortable, familiar environment.
      • Encourage the patient to invite a spouse, relative or friend, as appropriate.
      • Be adequately prepared regarding the clinical situation, being familiar with the patient's records and background.
      • Put aside your own baggage and personal feelings wherever possible.
   — Beginning the session/setting the scene
      • Summarise where things have got to and check with the patient.
      • Discover what has happened since last seen.
      • Calibrate how the patient is thinking/feeling.
      • Negotiate agenda.
   — Sharing the information
      • Assess the patient's understanding first: what the patient already knows, is thinking or has been told.
      • Gauge how much the patient wishes to know.
      • Give warning first that difficult information is coming, e.g. *I'm afraid we have some work to do . . . I'm afraid it looks more serious than we had hoped . . .*
      • Give basic information, simply and honestly; repeat important points.
      • Relate your explanation to the patient's perspective.
      • Do not give too much information too early; don't pussyfoot but do not overwhelm.
      • Give information in small chunks.
      • Watch the pace, check repeatedly for understanding and feelings as you proceed.
      • Use language carefully, taking into account the patient's intelligence, reactions and emotions, avoiding jargon.
      • Be aware of your own nonverbal behaviour throughout.
   — Being sensitive to the patient
      • Read and respond to the patient's non-verbal cues: face/body language, silences, tears.
      • Allow for 'shut down' (when patient turns off and stops listening) and then give time and space: allow possible denial.

- Keep pausing to give patient opportunity to ask questions.
- Gauge patient's need for further information as you go and give more information as requested, i.e. listen to the patient's wishes as patients vary greatly and one individual's preferences may vary over time or from one situation to another.
- Encourage the expression of feelings early, i.e. *How does that news leave you feeling?* or *I'm sorry that hearing this was difficult for you, you seem upset by that . . .*
- Respond to patient's feelings and predicament with acceptance, empathy and concern.
- Check patient's previous knowledge about information just given.
- Specifically elicit the patient's concerns.
- Check understanding of information given (*Would you like to run through what are you going to tell your son/parents/partner?*).
- Be aware of unshared meanings (i.e. what psychosis means for the patient compared with what it means for the clinician).
- Do not be afraid to show emotion or distress.

— Planning and support
- Having identified all the patient's specific concerns, offer specific help by breaking down overwhelming feelings into manageable concerns, prioritising and distinguishing the fixable from the unfixable.
- Identify a plan for what is to happen next.
- Give a broad time frame for what may lie ahead.
- Give hope tempered with realism, preparing for the worst and hoping for the best.
- Ally yourself with the patient, emphasising the partnership between clinician and patient (*We can work on this together . . . between us*), and confirming the role of the clinician as the advocate of the patient.
- Emphasise quality of life.
- Identify or create a safety net.

— Follow-up and closing
- Summarise and check with the patient and the family for understanding, offering space to ask additional questions.
- Don't rush the patient to treatment.
- Set up early further appointment, offer telephone calls, etc.
- Identify support systems; involve relatives and friends.
- Offer to see/tell relatives or others (e.g. partner, etc.).
- Make written materials available

— If the patient attends with family or a companion, read and respond to the other/s' verbal and non-verbal cues, allowing pauses for questions, but remember that the patient is your first concern.

— Throughout, be aware of your own anxieties around giving information, previous experience, and failure to cure or help.

3 List 10 aspects that you would take into consideration when breaking bad news to children or young people.

— How to break bad news to children and young people

- Adapt what you say to the child's age, developmental stage and level of understanding.
- Discuss with parents whether to tell the child, who should tell and what to tell. Respect parents' values; do not go over their heads.
- Try to learn what the child knows about the problems that s/he has.
- Be direct and honest. Avoid jargon. Do not lie. Do not give false reassurance.
- Give explanations in the presence of parents. Repeat information and check what the child has understood.
- Check what meaning the child attaches to explanations so as to avoid misunderstandings and unnecessary anxiety.
- Play, drawings, music, or psychotherapy sessions can help.
- Attend to needs and concerns of parents and siblings, who are sometimes more distressed than the child.
- Accept that a bad temper and tantrums are normal reactions in a severely ill child.
- Emphasise what the child will be able to do, thereby giving realistic hope.

OSCE model answer 14

Marking criteria

John will not be reassured by normal tests. If the doctor listens carefully, then he will open up and talk about when he was young.

He would really like to lead a normal life and doesn't know how to handle anxieties. He would like to work if he felt well. If the doctor sticks to their guns, he may begin to accept that it is not a good idea to have too many investigations because they can also carry a risk of causing more problems than they solve. He will feel relieved if the doctor listens attentively, and even though there may not be an answer, he will feel he could at least talk about his fears and that might help him control them. He might consider counselling or therapy if the doctor suggests it.

If the doctor keeps asking more physical questions, he will get more anxious and start wondering if there are more things wrong with him.

If the doctor talks too much and doesn't listen, he will not disclose as much and he will refuse a suggestion of counselling or therapy. If the doctor seems indecisive or nervous, he will lose confidence and question their competence and want to see another doctor.

Try to imagine someone else asking you questions about this patient. Do you really know him? Can you see how he comes to his own conclusions about his situation and his symptoms? If you can't answer the questions, you don't know enough yet. Even in short consultations, silence can be very helpful. Don't be tempted to focus into 'yes/no' questions until you are sure you have hit upon something worthwhile. If possible try to imagine and reflect his feelings.

Key points for model answer

➤ Introduces self, reason for consultation, confidentiality.
➤ Gathers background information, reason for consultations.
➤ Establishes patient's context, ideas, concerns and expectations.
➤ Listens attentively, using open questions and silences where necessary.
➤ Open body language and responds calmly to patient's anxiety.
➤ Explains tests were normal and that there is no need for further. investigations as they may cause more harm than good.
➤ Shared decision making around future management of anxiety, obsessional behaviour, enables patient to consider referral for therapy such as counselling, psychotherapy or CBT.

How not to do it:

1) John: *Do you really know what you're doing? You don't really seem to be sure. Could I see a consultant?*
   Dr: *We haven't found anything wrong so far. Do you have any other symptoms? Maybe we're missing something. I'll order a CT scan.*

2) John: *I went to a nutritionist. She told me I need a 'free T₃' test and that I'm intolerant to lots of foods. I've got this list, what do you think?*
   Dr: *It's probably rubbish. I'll refer you to the endocrinologist and gastroenterologist; that's the only way to get an accurate answer.*

3) John: *But doctors can miss cancer. I read it on the Internet; the government just wants to save money on tests.*
   Dr: *There's nothing wrong with you; there's nothing more I can do.*

4) John: *I just feel down because of these pains; I'm not depressed. Another doctor wanted to give me tablets but I didn't take them even when he gave me a prescription.*
   Dr: *I'll give you an antidepressant.*

These conversations cut off the possibility of exploring further what is troubling John and he may leave but will be unhappy, anxious and dissatisfied. He is likely to attend again, either with the same or another doctor. If the doctor behaves aggressively or negatively, the patient is likely to attend another doctor and begin the cycle again.

Try this instead:

Dr: *You look anxious. What are you thinking about?* (Responding to non-verbal cues and asking open questions.)

John: *I was always a worrier.*

Dr: *Tell me more.* (Open question.)

John: *My mum was on her own and I don't know much about my dad. I didn't have any brothers or sisters so mum worried about me. We worried about each other.*

Dr: How *did your mum cope with being alone?* (Recognising, validating, empathising.)

John: *Not very well, the house was a mess, she didn't always cook meals, sometimes I was hungry. We didn't have much money.*

Dr: *What about you?* (Recognising context, responding to verbal clues.)

John: *I was the neat one!*

Dr: *You tried to bring order into chaos?* (Suggested analysis.)

John: *Yes, I haven't thought of it like that before.*

Dr: *What happened when you were sick?* (Gathering information on child-hood history.)

John: *Mum always took me seriously if I got sick, she kept me off school and stayed with me.*

Dr: *How much time off did you have?* (Gather further information about impact on patient's life.)

John: *I did miss quite a bit of school. Nearly 18 months in all.*

Dr: *That's an unusually large amount of time. It must really have affected your education.* (Recognition and empathy.)

John: *Yes it did.*

Dr: *What did she do when you got sick, apart from keeping you at home?* (Gathering information.)

John: *She did take me to the doctor a few times.*

Dr: *What happened?*

John: *I had to have a few blood tests when I was feeling tired and ill after flu when I was 15. The blood test was a bit abnormal, I worried about it after that but the doctor said it was nothing to worry about.*

Dr: *It's been helpful hearing about your childhood experiences. Perhaps I could check a few other things, we may come back to that.* (Signposting.)

Do you mind telling me about your daily routine at the moment?

John: *I haven't got a job. I stay at home a lot.*

Dr: *That must be frustrating for you.* (Recognition, acknowledgement.)

John: *I want to work, I want to get out. But I worry. What if I have cancer or something else wrong, what if it's being missed? I try to keep clean, I wash my hands a lot to try to avoid catching things. I read you can catch viruses which cause cancer. That's true isn't it?*

Dr: *Sometimes we have to learn to manage not being sure about everything all the time. Why do you think that is hard for you?* (Explanation, attempt at hypothesis that this is harder for John than for others.)

John: *There was never much I could be sure about except that my mum did care about me.*

Dr: *Can I ask where your mother is now?* (Attempt to link past with present.)

John: *I live with her.* (New information the doctor did not previously know.)

Dr: *What's that like?* (Gathering information.)

John: (hesitates) . . . *Okay I suppose.*

Dr: *I'm wondering if you'd like to be more independent now? What would really help you make a change in your life?*

John: *Having a bit of money, having some friends.*

Dr: *Maybe no one has thought about helping you learn to cope with your feelings of anxiety about your health, maybe these stem from the stress and worry when you were young. Do you feel ready to move forward at all?* (Tentative suggested explanation of anxiety to patient. You may get clues about the origins of his anxieties. Try to imagine yourself in his shoes and the journey he has travelled in his life.)

John: *Maybe; but I'm not crazy, right?*

Dr: *No, I'm definitely not saying that* (responds to concern). *Your experiences in the past set up a pattern for your later life, maybe you learned some habits in the way you think about your health. We can help you to break those habits if you want to. For example, there are therapists who do something called cognitive behaviour therapy. They can help teach you ways of thinking and behaving differently.* (Suggested explanation and sharing ideas for further management. Don't make assumptions about what his mother did for him. This may yield vital clues, and the patient himself may never have articulated these feelings or thoughts before. The patient may not even realise they are repeating a pattern, or they may know it but need to say it.)

John: *I'd like to try something like that, but I'm afraid it might take up too much time and maybe I'm afraid my mum wouldn't cope without me if I left home.*

Dr: *So maybe you need to talk with her and maybe you both need help at the same time. Think about it. I can refer you anytime you feel ready.* (Responding to concerns, suggesting management solutions and allowing time to achieve a shared understanding.)

John: *Okay, thank you.*

Dr: *Why don't we meet again in 2 weeks' time when you've had a chance to talk to your mum and think about these ideas.* (Follow-up and support.)

John: *Thank you so much, I feel you've really understood me this time, doc. Goodbye.*

Dr: *Goodbye.* (Doctor feels sense of satisfaction with this consultation due to much better understanding of patient's context for the first time.)

Index

Entries in **bold** denote tables or figures.